Introduction to
Psychiatry

Introduction to Psychiatry

VMD Namboodiri

Consultant Psychiatrist
Sevana Hospital, Pattambi, Kerala

Former Head, Department of Psychiatry
MOSC Medical College and Hospital, Kolenchery
Kerala

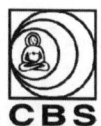

CBS

CBS Publishers & Distributors Pvt Ltd

New Delhi • Bengaluru • Chennai • Kochi • Kolkata • Mumbai
Bhopal • Bhubaneswar • Hyderabad • Jharkhand • Nagpur • Patna
• Pune • Uttarakhand • Dhaka (Bangladesh) • Kathmandu (Nepal)

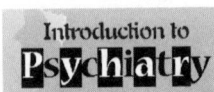

ISBN: 978-81-239-2399-4

Copyright © Author and Publisher

First Edition: 2014
Reprint: 2020

Published by Satish Kumar Jain and produced by Varun Jain for
CBS Publishers & Distributors Pvt Ltd
4819/XI Prahlad Street, 24 Ansari Road, Daryaganj, New Delhi 110 002, India.
Ph: 23289259, 23266861, 23266867   Fax: 011-23243014   Website: www.cbspd.com
e-mail: delhi@cbspd.com; cbspubs@airtelmail.in.

Corporate Office: 204 FIE, Industrial Area, Patparganj, Delhi 110 092
Ph: 011-4934 4934   Fax: 011-4934 4935   e-mail: publishing@cbspd.com;
                                                                    publicity@cbspd.com

Branches

- **Bengaluru:** Seema House 2975, 17th Cross, K.R. Road,
  Banasankari 2nd Stage, Bengaluru 560 070, Karnataka, India
  Ph: +91-80-26771678/79   Fax: +91-80-26771680   e-mail: bangalore@cbspd.com
- **Chennai:** 7, Subbaraya Street, Shenoy Nagar, Chennai 600 030, Tamil Nadu, India
  Ph: +91-44-26260666, 26208620   Fax: +91-44-42032115   e-mail: chennai@cbspd.com
- **Kochi:** 42/1325, 1326, Power House Road, Opp KSEB, Kochi 682 018, Kerala, India
  Ph: +91-484-4059061-65   Fax: +91-484-4059065   e-mail: kochi@cbspd.com
- **Kolkata:** 6/B, Ground Floor, Rameswar Shaw Road, Kolkata-700014 (West Bengal),
  India
  Ph: +91-33-2289-1126, 2289-1127, 2289-1128   e-mail: kolkata@cbspd.com
- **Mumbai:** 83-C, Dr E Moses Road, Worli, Mumbai-400018, Maharashtra, India
  Ph: +91-22-24902340/41   Fax: +91-22-24902342   e-mail: mumbai@cbspd.com

Representatives

• Bhopal	0-8319310552	• Bhubaneswar	0-9911037372	• Hyderabad	0-9885175004
• Jharkhand	0-9811541605	• Nagpur	0-9421945513	• Patna	0-9334159340
• Pune	0-9623451994	• Uttarakhand	0-9716462459	• Dhaka	01912-003485
• Kathmandu (Nepal)	977-9818742655			(Bangladesh)	

Printed at India Binding House, Noida, UP, India

Preface

This book, as its name suggests, is envisaged as a simple short introduction to the subject matter of psychiatry. Though primarily meant for the undergraduate students of medicine, the book would be useful to the students of clinical psychology, social work, and nursing as well. Description of most of the clinical conditions is supplemented by the case illustrations. The author believes that this will aid understanding.

I am grateful to Mr YN Arjuna for his interest and help in publishing this book without which the manuscript would not have seen light of the day. I also thank the entire editorial and production staff of CBS Publishers & Distributors for the fine preparation and production of the book.

Suggestions for improvement both in the contents and presentation are most welcome.

VMD Namboodiri

Contents

1

Scope of Psychiatry

The common man's concepts about psychiatry and its practitioners are rather fanciful. Unlike other medical conditions, the common man more often associates psychiatric disorders with culturally determined hypothetical causations which range from black magic to brain afflictions. All those who have a therapeutic alliance with the patient are indiscriminately called as psychiatrists, psychologists, psychotherapists or neurologists by convenience. Many people do not know the difference between a psychiatrist and a psychologist and a psychologist and a neurologist and their therapeutic roles. Many believe that a psychiatrist, or a psychologist for that matter, is a person who by looking at the patient's face can read his mind so as to later expurgate him of his "offensive thoughts" through "hypnotism" or through "talking out". Thus, while collecting details from a patient about his hallucinations I overheard the patient's father talking to his wife "see — doctor is taking out of Appu's mind all his bad thoughts"!

Elsewhere in some countries psychiatrists are fondly addressed as "head shrinkers". Psychiatrist is a person who treats "loonies" and the hospital for mentally ill is called a "loony bin". Even in our country the psychiatric patients have several pet names: "Half a screw less", "half a circle", or "full circle" (these depending on the degree of derangement), "crack", "nuts", "moonlight", etc. — people treating them also have similar endearing synonyms the exact terms varying from region to region.

A psychiatrist, or a psychologist has no mystical powers. As in any medical discipline he depends on the patient's history,

1

examination and investigations to arrive at a diagnosis. By definition a psychiatrist is a medical graduate who specializes in helping and treating people with emotional difficulties and disturbed interpersonal relationships as a result of their abnormal perceptions, feelings and thoughts. A medical background is essential for the therapist to comprehend the significance of the anatomical and physiological substrata of human behavior and to know how behavior is influenced by endogenous (meaning, generated inside the body) or exogenous (generated outside) chemical substances.

Reil and Psychiatry

The term psychiatry was first coined in 1808 by Johann Christian Reil (1759–1813), a German physician, anatomist and physiologist, famous for his discovery of the insula of the cerebral cortex ("The islands of Reil"). The term meant *"the soul as doctor"* (*iatros* = doctor) a way of treating the patient by using his *psyche* (meaning the soul) as the therapeutic agent. What he implied was that the *psyche* with its highly developed faculties like reasoning and judgement would help to cure insanity.

NORMAL AND ABNORMAL

It is often difficult to define what is normal behavior. It is more difficult to define its range—that is to say where normality ends and abnormality starts. What is considered as normal at one point of time may not be so at another epoch. It also varies with culture. In a country of cannibals a Buddhist monk preaching *ahimsa* (nonviolence) is as abnormal as a cannibal is in our midst. Certain behavior which is considered normal at one point of one's life may not be normal at another period. Examples are babbling and thumb sucking.

One important criterion of normal behavior is its social confirmity. This implies that in a given population a particular behavior which is shared by the majority of its members is accepted as normal. It is therefore a statistical criterion. Behavior which is deviant from the norms is a point of focus for the media also (Fig. 1.1).

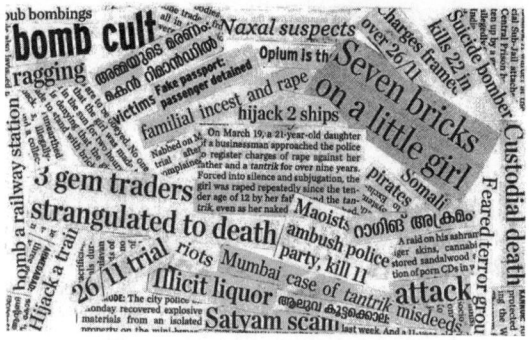

Fig. 1.1: Faces of abnormality

Though simple, statistical criterion will not by itself identify abnormality in many instances. As for example, consider the distribution of intelligence in a population. Most of its members fall within a particular range and qualify themselves as normal. But there are always a few who fall too low in their intelligence scores and also a few others who attain very high scores. Even though the former group alone may be considered as abnormal in a clinical setting both groups are qualified as abnormal according to the statistical norms as both groups deviate from the majority.

Another criterion which is considered in identifying abnormality is that of an "ideal state". Evidently this cannot be of any practical use as an ideal state, if at all present, is attainable only by a few persons thus disregarding the major bulk of the population.

In a clinical setting, the statistical criterion of abnormality is supplemented by another—presence of pathological symptoms which are a cause of distress either to the individual or to the community in which he lives. Thus the practical criteria of abnormal behavior include:

1. deviation from the social and statistical norms

2. personal misery (anxiety, fear, depression, etc.) and maladjustment

3. personal inefficiency and immaturity preventing the individual from fulfilling his expected role in the community.

CAUSES OF ABNORMALITY

It will be over simplifying to say that behavioral abnormalities are the resultant of one particular event. This is because of the multiplicity of causes which are constantly interacting and are also dynamic in nature. In psychiatry unlike in physical illnesses (even where the paradigm may fail), there is no one to one correlation between cause and effect. Even in physical illnesses (for example, a systemic infection), a number of factors affecting the invading organism's virulence and the host's vulnerability operate modifying the illness presentation.

Multiplicity of Factors

It is customary to categorize the etiological factors as biological, psychological and social (Table 1.1). The biological factors include heredity with its different modes of inheritance and constitutional factors like infection (e.g. encephalitis), trauma (e.g. head injury), metabolic causes (e.g. uremia), vascular causes (e.g. infarction), degeneration (e.g. senility), neoplasms (tumors), etc. The psychological factors include defective growth and personality development, poor coping skills, wrong attitudes, prejudices, etc. Social factors include pathological family environment, sibling and peer group rivalry, economic and cultural deprivations (due to factors related to race, religion, gender, etc.), migration, social catastrophies like war, famine and epidemics and others.

Interaction of Causes

The various etiological factors do not work in isolation but interact mutually and constantly — one influencing the other and being influenced by another. During this process, they assume the roles of predisposing and precipitating agents. The predisposing agents start working earlier and pave the way for further developments either compensatory or decompensatory The precipitating factors decide the epoch of disease manifestation by showing the symptoms. The precipitating causes of one instant may well be the predisposing factors of another instant and vice versa. Often the pattern of their interaction may be far from clear.

Table 1.1: Causes of abnormal behavior

FAULTY MAKE UP

Heredity
Infections and infestations
Trauma
Metabolic causes
Vascular causes
Degeneration
Neoplasms

FAULTY ENVIRONMENT

Family pathology
Sibling and peer group rivalry
Deprivation and bereavements
Unemployment
Economic instability
Marital disharmony
Social changes and insecurity
Migration
Catastrophic events

FAULTY ADJUSTMENT

Faulty learning
Poor coping skills
Inner conflicts
Frustrations
Prejudices

Dynamicity

The various etiological factors operate constantly and simultaneously. It is a dynamic process and the factors are not static. Some of them might have started operating even before the individual was born, say at the time of conception or while he was still in the mother's womb when they are qualified as hereditary or congenital respectively. After birth the individual continues to be influenced by them for the rest of his life. The disease is the end result of all such interactions and denote their combined effects on the individual and his adaptation to them—successful or not—at a particular time. Because of their nonstatic nature many use the term "dynamics of behavior" in preference to the word "etiology".

STRESS AND COPING

Stresses are the problems of adjustment operating at biological or psychosocial levels. Unless the individual adopts adjustive measures they may disturb the normal equilibrial state and the integrated functioning of the organism, this leading to pathological conditions.

Traffic accidents, infections, bodily afflictions, etc. are the examples of biological stresses. Sources of psychosocial stresses are frustrations, bereavements, conflicts, fear, anxiety, etc. Whenever there are stresses the body has inherent coping mechanisms to combat them. At a biological level compensatory mechanisms are mediated through the autonomic nervous system and the endocrine glands. Selye called this the General Adaptation Syndrome (GAS) and identified its three stages (Fig. 1.2), the alarm reaction, the stage of resistance and the stage of exhaustion. The third stage indicates that the organism is at the point of decompensation.

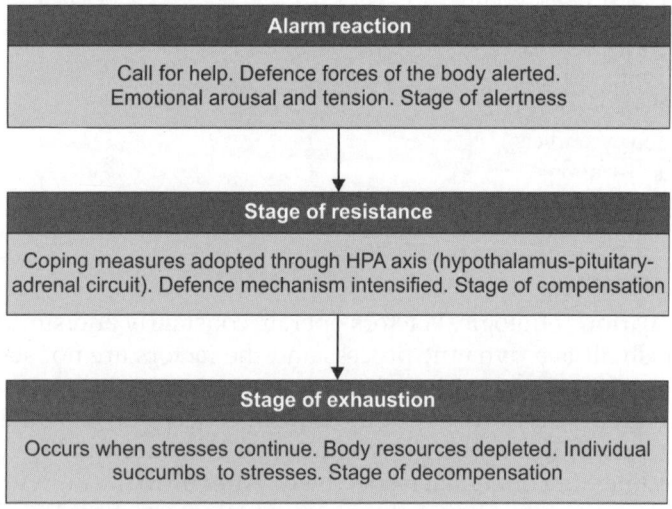

Fig. 1.2: General adaptation syndrome

DEFENCE MECHANISMS

As at the biological level there are coping mechanisms at a psychological level also which help to maintain the integrity of the self. Freud called them ego defence mechanisms as they are defences employed to protect "ego" or the conscious mind. The individual may not be aware of their presence as they operate at an "unconscious" level. Every individual at one time or other resorts to them. This is "normal" just as the biological ones are. Some of the important defence mechanisms are the following:

i. **Denial:** Among the defence mechanisms denial is the simplest and the most primitive one. Here, the individual avoids an unpleasant reality by ignoring its presence. Thus one who has a life-threatening disease of which he is aware belittles its seriousness by "forgetting" to take the medicines in time or to see the doctor regularly. Those who are afraid of death and its inevitability wears a seemingly resigned attitude and makes casual remarks as "death is inevitable" or "all those born shall die one day". The alcoholic denies his illness by believing that he has no serious problem as he drinks only in the evenings and not regularly.

ii. **Repression:** Thoughts, experiences or impulses invoking guilt feelings and which on retrospect produce shame and self reproach are pushed into "unconscious" through repression. When successfully repressed these feelings are denied access to consciousness. The individual "forgets" such painful events selectively and is unable to recall them by his conscious efforts. A person who loses all his belongings in a social riot, and who had to flee from his home may not even remember that there was a riot. One who is jealous of his colleague who is admittedly smarter than him "represses" his jealousy and assumes an extra cordial relationship with him (this known as reaction formation in psychology).

Repressed material does not remain dormant in the unconscious for long. It tries to enter the conscious realm through slips of tongue, "accidental" acts of the individual the purpose of which he does not know or through his dreams. It may produce "conversion symptoms" where a mental conflict is "converted" to a physical symptom (for example "hysterical" blindness).

iii. **Sublimation:** Sublimation is the process of channeling out ungratified desires and impulses to socially accepted activities. Thus, the woman denied of a maternal role due to failed marriage finds happiness in working for child welfare.

iv. **Rationalization:** In simple language, rationalization is "giving bad reasons for what we do on impulse". One hunts for arguments to justify his action and after finding them convinces himself that it was the real motive for his action. Going back to the alcoholic what all excuses does he find each time to justify his temptations! It is a new brand; it is a sin to waste as the glass was already filled. It is a social obligation; it would be an insult to his companions if he did not join them; it was a special occasion; it helps him to concentrate or to relax; it is only once this time and one does not matter; or it helps him to take a resolve not to touch it again. Countries go to war "not to grab the other country's land and resources" but because "they want to help the people in that country to set a model government".

v. **Projection:** In this mechanism, the individual projects his shortcomings and objectionable qualities (which he refuses to accept as having) on others and blames them for having these qualities. The greedy accuse others of greed. The student who fails in the examination believes that his teachers were unfair and failed him. Often the objects of projection are fate and bad luck—as "he would have succeeded if the providence was not against him".

vi. **Phantasy:** In plain language, phantasy is day dreaming. It is a mechanism universally resorted to when desires are thwarted. It is a retreat from the real world to an imaginary world where his needs are gratified and desires fulfilled. The mediocre student has phantasies of coming out in the exams in flying colors. The half starved man phantasies himself to be in a feast hall.

There are several other mental mechanisms which are resorted to for coping up stresses. As mentioned earlier, the individual may not be aware of the nature or even the presence of a stress. Similarly, the coping up mechanisms also may operate at a conscious or unconscious level. Stress arouses various emotions—fear, or anxiety or anger and the subject may be aware of these emotional accompaniments only. In all cases the whole individual, not a part of it, reacts to the stress— physically and psychologically, that is the reactions are holistic. The reactions are also economical with the minimum expenditure of energy as possible so as not to deplete him of his resources unnecessarily.

The individual's tolerance to stress (or frustration) varies considerably. This partly depends on the severity of stress. Stresses are severe when they are long standing, multiple or repetitive. But it is the subjective evaluation of the stress or the importance attached to the problem by the individual which is crucial in deciding the severity of the stress.

When the coping mechanisms fail or decompensate either due to the severity of stress or the individual's poor stress tolerance the organism breaks down leading to various morbid conditions.

PATTERNS OF ILLNESS

These vary widely and are discussed in greater detail in the subsequent chapters.

Psychosis and Neurosis

Psychosis (pl. psychoses), neurosis (pl. nuroses), and their adjectival forms psychotic and neurotic are the terms which are very frequently used in psychiatry. Psychosis refers to a group of disorders which are severe and disabling due to their gross distortion of mental functioning. Distortion of mental functions occur at several levels.

Confusion and other disturbances of sensorium	Cause disturbances in attending to reality (meaning the real world)
Hallucinations	Cause disturbances in perceiving reality
Delusions	Cause disturbances in interpreting reality
Social withdrawal	Cause disturbances in interacting with reality

Because of these gross impairments, the psychotic has severe problems in relating to his environment and people around. He lives in a world of phantasy created from his misperceptions and misinterpretations believing that it is the real world and that his experiences are shared by others also. Look at the following example.

CASE 1

Sam, 23-year-old, went to Bangalore to attend an interview for a tool designer's post. Just before reaching the city he was woken up from his reverie by a male voice calling his name repeatedly. He looked around to find the source of the sound and discovered that it was coming from outside, outside the running bus, from near the window pane. The voice asked him not to attend the interview and to return home. Sam wondered what was happening when the voice ("reading my thoughts") explained that the interview was a hoax for recruiting young men who would be sent abroad and their heart and kidneys removed. The voice warned Sam to keep away from a man "in a red checked shirt" who was the pin of the racket. Reaching Bangalore Sam was afraid to get down from the bus because of the "man in the red checked shirt." He did not call his parents in Kerala nor his relatives in Bangalore to report of his arrival in the city. Also he did not attend the interview. After a frantic search for three days by the anxious relatives and with police help Sam was found hiding in an abandoned railway coach starving and emaciated, deprived of money and all his belongings. He did not dare to step out as "people were waiting to catch and hand him over to the man in the red shirt".

Some other features of psychosis are: (i) incoherent speech which results from disturbances of thinking. Thinking is fragmented and it has no direction. It may also get blocked in between, (ii) prolonged and excessive melancholy or exhilaration, (iii) grossly impaired memory, and (iv) severely disturbed social and personal functioning.

In neurosis on the other hand the individual retains contact with reality as his perceptions and interpretations are not distorted with hallucinations and delusions. The characteristic symptom of neurosis is anxiety which signifies mental conflicts and maladaptive responses to stress. Symptoms like "worry", "irritability", "tension", etc. are indicators of anxiety. "Forgetting" and obsessional thoughts and rituals indicate self-defeating attempts of the individual to overcome anxiety whereas "depression" and fatigue are the residuals of prolonged tension. The individual is distressingly aware of his symptoms and recognizes them as irrational and pathological (ego alien) unlike a psychotic.

Organic Mental Disorders

The term organic is used to distinguish a group of disorders in which there is evidence of brain dysfunction causing or modifying the patient's symptoms. The dysfunction may be primary as when the brain is affected directly. Examples are trauma (e.g. head injury), infections (e.g. encephalitis), vascular (e.g. cerebral thrombosis), toxemias (e.g. drug intoxication), neoplasms (e.g. tumors of brain), degeneration (e.g. dementia), etc. It may be secondary as when brain is affected subsequent to a disease process elsewhere in the body. Uremia is an example.

The most remarkable features of an organic mental disorder are disturbances of consciousness, attention, memory, learning and intellect. However, there are instances where these functions are spared and instead disturbances of perception, thinking, feeling or general behavior are manifested as the presenting symptoms. The symptoms differ depending on their duration also. That is, the features of an acute organic disorder are entirely different from those of a chronic one.

Organic mental disorders may be psychotic or non-psychotic. In the former because of the perceptual and other disturbances the individual loses his capacity to relate normally to the environment as occurs in delirium. In the latter this capacity is retained. An example is sleep disorders due to organic causes.

Personality Disorders

Personality disorders are patterns of maladaptive behavior which produce personal distress, or impairment of social functioning or both. Unlike psychoses and neuroses which are time limited syndromes (having a beginning and an end), personality disorders are lifelong patterns which manifest as early as adolescence or early adulthood. They are also not limited to any one area of special functioning like cognition or mood, that is they are pervasive affecting all areas of the individual's personality. Several clinically diverse conditions which are described in the later chapters are included in this category.

CLASSIFICATION

Classification is categorizing disorders into groups and subgroups based on the similarities shared by all members of that group. There are various ways of classification, just as there are various ways of arranging things spread on a desktop. Classifying diseases according to their etiology is one way and sorting them depending on the clinical features is another. In psychiatry, disorders are mostly classified according to their symptoms and the course of illness.

Classification serves several useful purposes. The important ones are: (i) order and compactness of data, (ii) easy communication, (iii) research and education, (iv) administration, (v) legal purposes. There are two prevalent systems of classification in psychiatry. They are the ICD (International Classification of Mental and Behavioural Disorders) produced by WHO and the DSM (Diagnostic and Statistical Manual of Mental Disorders) published by the American Psychiatric Association. In India international classification is the official diagnostic system.

International Classification

According to the International Classification of Mental and Behavioural Disorders (ICD-10, meaning 10th revision) published by the World Health Organisation in 1992, chapter V (designated by the letter F) is exclusively devoted to psychiatric disorders. There are 10 blocks (F0–F9) each with 10 categories. For example, F0 has 10 categories from F00 to F09. The 10 categories of F9 are F90 to F99. Thus there are altogether 100 categories (F00, F01, F02.... F09, F10, F11 ... F19, F20... F99) to list mental and behavioral disorders. The first digit after the letter F denotes the main category of a disorder (Table 1.2).

Table 1.2: Main categories of mental and behavioral disorders according to ICD–10

Category	Disorder
F0	Organic, including symptomatic mental disorders
F1	Mental and Behavioural disorders due to psychoactive substance use
F2	Schizophrenia, schizotypal and delusional disorders
F3	Mood (affective) disorders
F4	Neurotic, stress related and somatoform disorders
F5	Behavioral syndromes associated with physiological disturbances and physical factors
F6	Disorders of adult personality and behavior
F7	Mental retardation
F8	Disorders of psychological development
F9	Behavioral and mental disorders with onset usually occurring in childhood and adolescence

i. **Organic mental disorders (F00–F09):** Mental disorders due to cerebral dysfunction are listed in this group. Brain may be affected primarily or secondarily. The various dementias, deliriums and other behavioral disorders like anomalies of perception, mood, thinking and personality due to organic causes are included in this category.

ii. **Disorders due to substance use (F10–F19):** This category lists disorders consequent to the use of psychoactive substances like alcohol, opium, cannabis, etc.

iii. **Schizophrenia, schizotypal and delusional disorders (F20–F29):** The different types of schizophrenia, as well as schizophrenia like conditions and conditions where paranoid symptoms are most prominent are included in this category.

iv. **Mood disorders (F30–F39):** The basic disturbance in this group of disorders is morbid alterations of mood—depression and elation with or without psychotic symptoms. There will be associated disturbances of activity and thinking which are secondary to the mood change.

v. **Neurotic disorders (F40–F49):** This category includes the different neurotic disorders like phobias, anxiety disorders, obsessive compulsive disorder and dissociative (conversion disorders). In addition, it includes reactions to stress and somatoform disorders characterized by intense preoccupation with bodily symptoms.

vi. **Behavioral disturbances associated with physiological and physical disturbances (F50–59):** This is a wide group of disorders related to eating (e.g. anorexia), sleep (insomnia, hypersomnia, nightmares, etc.) and sexual functioning (e.g. frigidity, premature ejaculation). It also includes disturbances seen in the post-partum period and those following harmful use of certain drugs like laxatives, analgesics, steroids, etc.

vii. **Adult personality disorders (F60-F69):** This comprises specific personality disorders and habit and impulse disorders as were mentioned earlier. In addition disturbances related to sexual orientation (e.g. homosexuality) and preference (e.g. exhibitionism) are coded here.

viii. **Mental retardation (F70–79):** Various degrees of mental retardation (mild, moderate, severe and profound) are listed in this category.

ix. **Disorders of psychological development (F80–F89):** Specific developmental disorders like language disorders and disorders of reading, spelling, arithmetical skill, etc.) and pervasive developmental disorders (e.g. childhood autism) are listed in this block.

x. **Disorders with onset in childhood (F90–F98):** Some disorders which are first noted in infancy and childhood are included here. These include conditions like hyperkinetic disorders, conduct and emotional disorders of childhood, tic disorders, enuresis, encopresis, feeding disorders, pica, stammering, etc.

Some Subspecialities in Psychiatry

Addiction psychiatry
Specifically deals with problems related to addiction and addicts. Addiction by one definition is continued use of psychoactive substances despite physical, psychological and social harm.

Child and adolescent psychiatry
Speciality dealing with problems related to childhood and adolescence.

Community psychiatry
Psychiatric practice in the open community as against in a formal hospital setting.

Forensic psychiatry
Legal psychiatry is a subspeciality concerned with application of psychiatry for legal purposes. It deals with legal issues in which the psychiatric patient is involved.

Geriatric psychiatry
Study of psychological aspects of aging and specific psychiatric problems encountered by elderly people.

Liaison psychiatry
Deals with matters related to practice of psychiatry in a general hospital setting where the psychiatrist works in liaison with other medical specialists.

Military psychiatry
Speciality dealing with psychiatric problems in relation to military service and personnel.

Social psychiatry
Psychiatric speciality concerned with the effect of human environment on mental illness.

THERAPEUTIC TEAM IN PSYCHIATRY

Psychiatric disorders are complex and require a multi-disciplinary approach and treatment team. Its members are specialists in their respective fields. With team work there is pooling of skills which improves the quality of patient care. Team members have their goals defined but they work interdependently to achieve the common purpose. Table 1.3 lists the important and most essential members of the team.

Table 1.3: Team work in Psychiatry — Members of the therapeutic team

Psychiatrist

Medical graduate (MBBS) with post graduate specialization in psychiatry (DPM, Dip NB, MD). Psychiatrists alone are licensed to prescribe medicines and to carry out other methods of somatic treatment.

Clinical psychologist

Non-medical therapist with a basic postgraduate degree in psychology (MA/MSc) and specialization in clinical psychology (MPhil/PhD). They administer the various psychological tests in addition to carrying out psychosocial methods of treatment.

Psychiatric social worker

Graduate in psychology or social work with postgraduate training in psychiatric social work. Besides carrying out some psychosocial methods of treatment, they assess and help to rectify faults in the patient's home and work environments. Also in liaison with community's social agencies they help to rehabilitate the patient.

Psychiatric nurse

Graduate nurse with postgraduate training in psychiatric nursing. In addition to dispensing medicines and care giving, she keeps patients under constant observation, particularly those who have specific problems (suicidal risk, aggression, self neglect, etc.). She also takes part in the group therapeutic programs conducted inside the hospital.

Occupational therapist

Graduates or postgraduates in occupational therapy (DOT/BOT/MOT). After assessment of a patient the occupational therapist selects a craft which is most suited for the patient's physical and psychological rehabilitation. Occupational therapy is often combined with recreational activities. New skills are learnt, self-confidence and competitiveness are enhanced and interaction with others is strengthened by occupational therapy.

Psychiatric aides

Male or female members of the nursing staff. They do not have a professional qualification as a nurse but are imparted orientation courses in ongoing in-service programmes and individual supervision by a qualified staff nurse. They assist nurses in caring to the physical needs of the patient (feeding, dressing, etc.).

2

Symptoms and Signs

Cognition, conation and emotion are usually considered as the functions of the mind. Roughly translated they mean: knowing (the world), willing (to act) and feeling. In disorders of the mind, these faculties are deranged and the patient presents with symptoms referable to their defective functioning. The commonly encountered dysfunctions of mind are enumerated in this chapter.

COGNITIVE DISORDERS

Cognition involves several processes. They are attending, perceiving, learning and thinking. Defects may occur at each level.

DISORDERS OF ATTENTION

Attention is the ability to focus selectively on a particular task or activity. Concentration is sustaining that focus or "sustained or focused attention". Distraction is the inability to shut off irrelevant stimuli. Divided attention is attending to two stimuli alternatingly.

Disorders of attention occur in a variety of psychiatric conditions, both organic and functional as well as psychotic and neurotic. Hence, it has no diagnostic value. Attention is altered in altered physiological states, as, for example fatigue and tiredness.

DISORDERS OF PERCEPTION

Perception is defined as "the process of organizing and interpreting sensory data by combining them with results of past experience." Sensory data produced as a result of stimulation of end organs or receptors are unqualified and become meaningful in the light of past experience. The implications are that there is no perception if there are no sensory data or past experience or when they are not integrated (combined).

Perceptual disorders are mainly two—illusions and hallucinations.

Illusions

Illusions are false perceptions of a real object. They are misinterpretations of a real object, when the external stimuli are diminished, as for example, dimness of light. In fading light a rope is taken for a snake. It also occurs when the sensorium of the observer is clouded—as in delirium or confusion. Some mental states (e.g. fear, anxiety) worsen them further. Illusions occur in all sensory fields and are named accordingly.

Box 2.1: Illusions

Illusions are false perceptions of a real object. If a spoon is partially immersed in a glass of water the submerged portion appears to be bent. This is an illusion. In the fading light a rope is misjudged as a snake. Marks on the wall look like crawling insects. The silhouette of a tree trunk is taken for a lurking human figure. All these are examples of optical illusions.

Illusions occur in all sensory fields. Many of them are "normal", meaning they reflect the integrity of our perception and pervade our day to day life. The moon illusion is an age old phenomenon. The sun and moon appear much larger at the horizon than at zenith — even though infact they are of the same size. We all believe that the figure 3 and 8 (and the letters B, K, E, S, etc.) have two equal halves. But they do not have. To prove this turn the book upside down and see that their upper half is smaller than the lower one.

The proofreader's illusion

The proofreader's illusion can be convniently grouped along with. The proof reading essentially should be a slow proess to minmize possbilities of skippng over wrongly prnted words. It is somtimes fantastic how many mispelt words escape their (and ours too) attntion. More than half the words of the text are subtituted from the proofreader's mind. Chidren not old enogh to perceve wrds at a glance commit lesser mistkes (incidentally you were also subjected to the same illusion if any of the 18 mistakes in this paragraph escaped your attention).

Hallucinations

Hallucinations are false perceptions in the absence of an external object. Like illusions they may occur in any sensory modality and are named accordingly. Ordinarily hallucinations are the hall mark of psychoses but they may occur in "normal" conditions also — as prior to waking up (hypnapompic) and before sleeping (hypnagogic). Though commonly visual, they can occur in other sensory modalities also.

Hallucinations are classified depending on several characteristics (Table 2.1).

Special Types of Hallucinations

Extracampine: Hallucinations are called extracampine when they occur outside the ordinary limits of sense perception. Examples are: hearing conversation taking place several kilometers away, being able to see through the top of one's head, etc.

Reflex hallucinations (synesthesiae): Two sensory modalities are involved here. Stimulation of one sense modality gives sensory data pertaining to the other, as for example, "hearing" colors, "seeing" music. Synesthesiae are common in intoxications particularly due to LSD and other similar psychomimetic agents.

Table 2.1: Classification of hallucinations	
Characteristics	*Classification*
Depending on the sensory modality	Auditory, visual, tactile, etc.
Depending on the reality value	True hallucinations and false (pseudo) hallucinations
Depending on the complexity	Simple (elemental) e.g. flashes of light, tapping sound and complex (when several sense modalities are involved) e.g. a wildfire where visual (tongues of flame), auditory (crackling wood) and olfactory (smoke) sense modalities are involved
Depending on the organization	Formed (voices) and unformed (noises)
Special types	Extracampine, reflex hallucinations, functional, etc.

Functional hallucinations: Here stimulation of one sensory modality provokes another and both are heard at the same time, as, for example, bird chirps and the person hears human voices or the fan revolves and patient hears his name being called.

OTHER PERCEPTUAL DISTURBANCES

Sensory Distortions

These occur in all sense modalities and refer to changes in intensity and quality. Sounds become louder and colors brighter in hyperesthesia. They fade or lose color in hypoaesthesia. Sensations become perverted or distorted in paresthesia. Hyperesthesia occurs under intense emotional states, acute psychoses and prior to epileptic seizures. Hypoesthesia occurs in depression and delirium and more intense stimulation is needed to arouse him. Sensations are distorted under effects of psychedelic drugs.

Perceptual Disturbances of Time and Space

Perception of time and space differs from others in that they lack any special sense organs. Time and space are eternal and *pervade* all life activities. They serve as reference grids to our life activities and are perceived along with them. They are linked with all sensory processes and never *vanish*. The extent, duration and mode of experiencing them alone are modified. Thus, time stands still or its passage is too slow when engaged in a dull, monotonous activity or in depression and anxiety. Each minute appears as long as an age. In contrast time moves fast in mania and in intoxications or while indulging in an interesting activity. Time is experienced as a continuous flow with no "gaps" in between. This is lost in schizophrenia where "gap of emptiness" fall in between two points of experience.

Space appears large and boundless in disturbances of space. Things appear small and far away (micropsia) or large and near (macropsia).

Disturbances of Body Image

Autoscopy: In autoscopy one's own body is projected in external space and is found floating in front of him. This occurs in certain intoxications (e.g. ketamine) and in near death experience (NDE). He may be looking upon his own lifeless body lying on the cot, as he reports after wards.

Phantom limb: Even after a limb is amputated or a body part removed, the patient feels its "real" existence and all sensations including pain.

In organic lesions of the brain there are disturbances of body image like right/left disorientation, anosognosia (ignoring the presence of illness—like paralysis) and autotopagnosia (inability to recognise one's own body parts). Alterations of bodily experience occur in nonorganic conditions also. The body may appear shrivelled up and misshapen and body parts are displaced or duplicated.

Percepts and Memory Images

Percepts are units of perception. They differ from memory images. The differences are given in Table 2.2.

DISORDERS OF LEARNING (MEMORY)

Memory involves the capacity to register, retain and recall images, ideas or concepts. Disturbance at each level interferes with learning. Defects in registration occur when the stimuli are weak or inadequate or when the subject's sensorium is not clear (e.g. intoxicated states). Defects in retention occur when the memory traces fade out, as for example, lack of practice. Defects of recall occur when the preceding stages are faulty. All the three types may occur due to organic lesions or under emotional turmoil.

Table 2.2: Percepts and memory images	
Percepts	*Memory images*
1. Occur in external space	Occurs in internal space ("the mind")
2. Has no voluntary control	Can be retrieved and terminated at will
3. Appear true and life like	Subject is aware that the image is virtual
4. Remain constant and unchanged	Fade off over time like memory

Disorders of memory present as amnesias, hypermnesias and paramensias.

Amnesias

Amnesia is the inability to recollect past happenings. It may be (a) partial or total or (b) specific (e.g. learning numbers) or general. Amnesia can also be for immediate events (e.g. repetition of a series of numbers), recent (a few minutes to a few hours) or remote events. A brain injury causing loss of consciousness may be related temporally to amnesia. Loss of memory for events that occurred prior to the lesion is called retrograde amnesia as against anterograde amnesia which occurs following the lesion.

Amnestic syndrome is impaired memory for recent and remote events, where the subject is in clear consciousness. It is commonly seen in Korsakov's psychosis due to chronic alcoholism. There is associated confabulation (see below) and difficulty in learning new material.

Hypermnesia

In hypermnesia, there is an extreme degree of correct recall of past events. Even trivial details are remembered accurately. This is commonly seen in hypomania, delusional disorders and obsessive compulsive disorders.

Paramnesias

Paramnesias are unintentional falsification or distortion of events either in detail or in their temporal relationships.

Confabulation

Confabulation is the unintentional filling of memory gaps with material which are false and fanciful. Such recalls may change from moment to moment.

deja vu is an error of recognition where events though occurring for the first time appear to have happened earlier. The subject feels that he is reliving the experience.

In contrast *jamais vu* is the feeling of total strangeness to familiar objects and events.

DISORDERS OF THOUGHT

Ability to think and use language crowns man's mental faculties. Man alone is called *"homo sapiens"* (thinking animal) because of this ability. Thinking involves abstraction, concept formation and symbolization.

Disorders of thought are mainly three:
1. disorders of form
2. disorders of progression and
3. disorders of content

Formal Thought Disorders

Disordered forms of thought present as various logical and syntactical errors and errors of abstraction and conceptualization. The common errors are the following:

Autistic Thinking

Autism refers to an extreme degree of preoccupation with fantasies, hallucinations and delusions so that touch with reality is lost. An example is a patient who believes that he can weave invisible clothes by using moon's rays.

Incoherence

The usual association between one idea and the succeeding one is lost. Talk becomes a jumble of confused ideas with no connecting links between them. In extreme cases, the language assumes the form of a jargon when the term "word salad" is used, as an example may be quoted *"soldiers come about three red months April to rain and ordered to shoot"*. New words may be coined (Neologism) which bears no meaning except to the patient. As, for example, one patient repeatedly used the word *"doondle"* when he was asked where his house was. According to the patient the word meant down the hill where his house really situated. Another patient (a clerk in a bank) used the word *"compost"* to mean compound interest.

Concretism

Concretism refers to lack of abstraction and inability to form concepts. Thus a patient interpreted the common usage "green with envy" to indicate that the person virtually became green in color.

Illogical Thinking

The thought becomes totally illogical as when a patient remarked "Mother wears a white saree. Sita wears white saree. So Sita is my mother".

Disorders of Progression

Disorders of progression are seen at three levels—pace, volume and direction.

Disorders of Pace

The pace may be slow as in depression and the patient takes unduly long time to speak or reply to questions. The thought stream may stop suddenly. This is known as thought block and occurs in schizophrenia. In contrast, in mania or psychomotor excitement the patient speaks fast to the extent of even incoherence due the speed (flight of ideas). Rhyming and punning are other examples of progression. In rhyming the intended word is replaced by another word which sounds similar like sound and hound or head and bread. Instead of telling a loaf of bread he may say a loaf of head. Punning is a humorous play with the words which sound similarly but again have different meanings. An example is: *seven days with no food make one weak (weak/week).*

Volume

In poverty of speech there is paucity of ideas as against in verbigeration where there is excessive production.

Direction

In circumstantiality there is undue elaboration of details and the main point is reached subsequently after inclusion of irrelevant details in its course. In another form of direction the goal is not reached, the talk being sidetracked more and more from the main theme. This is called tangentiality. Examples of the two are given as follows.

Circumstantiality

Q. Why did you come to the hospital?

A. "That exactly is the point. When I received the phone call from my uncle yesterday I decided to call my brother. He had been away for the week end and came back today morning only. He has a car, you see, got it secondhand from his friend in Palakkad. We set together by car to see you".

Tangentiality

Q. Why did you come to the hospital?

A. "I was planning to come here last week. Last week was my son's birthday. Several people had come home and there was Ramakumar also. He works in Delhi on a contract basis. It is unduly hot in Delhi now and you can't think of settling there because of the high cost of living".

Disorders of Content

The main disorders belonging to this category are the delusions. Delusions are false beliefs which have no bearing with reality and are fixed and unchangeable even with logical reasoning. They are not shared by other members of population and do not agree with one's level of education or knowledge. An example is a patient's conviction that the CIDs have planted electronic gadgets in his body to spy on him.

Delusions are of several types. The common themes of delusions are the following.

Persecutory Delusions

The patient believes that he is harassed or persecuted by his enemies. The above example of CIDs? harassing him by implanting electronic gadgets in his body represents a persecutory delusion. Other examples are false beliefs that he is being poisoned or harmed through black magic, X-rays or physical force.

Grandiose Delusion

These are false and exalted beliefs of self importance, having beliefs that he is endowed with superhuman powers, money or other accomplishments. He might believe that he is the "chosen one" or leader born to carry out a special mission.

Delusions of Infidelity

These often occur among marital partners, one accusing the other of being unfaithful and indulging in extramarital relationships.

Delusions of Sin and Guilt

Here, the patient believes that he is the worst sinner and reproaches himself for his "bad deeds" bringing calamity to people around him. An example is one patient's belief that his past sins caused floods in the state.

Nihilistic Delusions

The patient holds that his body and organs are rotten and that he is no more alive.

Delusions of Reference

All happenings around him are interpreted as directed at him, that people are talking about him or making remarks at him.

Hypochondriacal Delusions

Here the theme is one of ill health. The patient believes that he has a serious or incurable illness like cancer or AIDS which the doctors have failed to detect.

Delusions are said to be systematized when they are fully developed and made seemingly "logical" and coherent. They are said to be mood congruent when delusions are keeping harmony with the prevailing mood. A manic patient who believes that people are jealous of him because of his superior accomplishments is an example. A delusion which is not in keeping with his mood is called mood incongruent.

Box 2.2: Illusions, Hallucinations and Delusions

Many a time these three words are wrongly used or interchanged. Both illusion and hallucinations are errors of perception occurring at the time of handling the sensory data. Presence of an actual stimulus differentiates illusions from hallucinations. Delusion on the other hand is a disorder of thinking, a fixed false incorrigible belief which occurs at a higher level of the cognitive process. Using the earlier example it is called an illusion when the rope is mistaken for a snake. It becomes a hallucination when the person "sees" a snake when there is neither a rope nor a snake. It is named a delusion when the person firmly believes and alleges that there is a snake around when infact it is not present.

Obsessions and Phobias

Obsessions are recurrent ideas or images or impulses that intrude the person's mind again and again which he tries to resist without success. Unlike delusions obsessions are "ego alien" meaning that the person considers them as strange, irrational and repulsive. Phobias are exaggerated and morbid fears of a neutral stimulus or situation which the person avoids because of the dread. They can occur in a variety of situations, like closed spaces, heights or crowded streets. Both obsession and phobia occur against a person's will and in spite of willful efforts to avoid them they invade his mind causing distress and agony.

VOLITIONAL (MOTOR) DISTURBANCES

Motor disturbances could be signs of an organic illness, though all of them are not of neurological origin. In such cases they are disturbances of volition, i.e disturbances of will and can be broadly divided into three types:

1. Akinetic states

2. Hyperkinetic states

3. Parakinetic states

Akinetic States

They are characterized by slowness and under—activity, including psychomotor retardation. Movements are slow and strained and speech is minimal. Level of activity is reduced and in its severe form they present as stupor characterized by akinesia (loss of movement), mutism and autonomic nervous dysfunction as, for example, urinary incontinence. In stupor, the patient is totally immobile, though he may be in touch with his surroundings as he reports retrospectively. Stupor may be due to schizophrenia, depression, dissociation disorder or an organic illness. In organic stupor, however, the level of consciousness is altered.

Hyperkinetic States

They are characterized by hyperactivity and psychomotor acceleration. Hyperactivity may be goal directed or not. In mania they appear to be goal directed but the goal is not reached due to intervening distracting stimuli. In schizophrenia the excitement is bizarre and the acts purposeless. At times the acts are impulsive. Depressed patients sometimes become restless and agitated which resembles excitement. Excitement may be organic in origin as in delirium or epilepsy.

Parakinetic States

Stereotypy is persistent repetition of words, gestures or movements which are not goal directed and are carried out uniformly without any external stimulus.

Perseveration is continuation of a goal directed response even after its purpose is fulfilled. The patient is unable to stop it. It is a common feature of frontal lobe dysfunction and is organic in origin.

Waxy flexibility is maintenance of a particular posture for long periods of time. The posture may be bizarre and uncomfortable, imposed on the patient by the examiner which the patient continues to maintain.

Echopraxia and Echolalia

Echopraxia is repetition of movements carried out by the examiner. In *echolalia* the patient repeats words spoken by the examiner.

Negativism and Automatism

Negativism is resistance to all passive movements or commands. The patient refuses to carry out even small commands (as for example, showing the tongue). In automatism all commands are passively carried out without regard to their consequences.

Ambivalence is simultaneous, contradictory feelings or actions toward the same object which do not reach the intended goal, as for example the patient extends his hands towards the examiner, but suddenly withdraws them and extends again as if for shaking hands.

DISORDERS OF MOOD

Feeling, affect, mood and emotion are all terms to indicate the feeling tone and are often used interchangeably. Emotion is the stirred up state because of the physiological changes which accompany an experience. Affects are waves of emotion that surf up periodically for short periods of time. Affect sustained for a long period is called the mood. Feeling is the subjective experience of emotion.

Abnormality of emotions present as their abnormal presence, duration and depth, fluctuations and appropriateness. Fear, anxiety, depression, anger, etc. are the examples of abnormal presence. Emotions are abnormal when they are out of proportion to the event and when they persist for unduly long periods even after the event is over

Lability of emotions refers to rapid fluctuation, say from joy to sorrow and anger. Extreme variation is called incontinence. Reduced expression of emotions is called flattening or bluntness and its extreme form is called apathy.

Mood is called inappropriate when it is not in tune with the circumstances, as for example, feeling happy when there is a loss and where the situation warrants sadness. Mood is a subjective state but objective evaluation is often possible by the physiological accompaniments of the emotion.

Anxiety is an unpleasant state of expectation of any untoward happening without the certainty of its happening. Fear implies a real threat and is related to an external object. Depression is feeling of sadness, usually a reaction to a loss, real or imagined. The opposite is elation, a feeling of undue happiness which in progressively more severe degrees are called euphoria, exaltation and ecstasy. Anger is strong and sometimes violent feelings of displeasure. Apathy refers to "lack of feeling", a total indifference to the feeling.

OTHER PRESENTING SYMPTOMS

Disturbances of Consciousness

Consciousness is awareness of self and environment. Its level varies from full alertness to coma with intervening stages of confusion and stupor. *Confusion* is an inability to think clearly. *Stupor* is a state of impaired consciousness, where the patient can be aroused with difficulty only. Compare this with stupor in psychiatry. Stupor in psychiatry refers to a state of immobility, irresponsiveness to environment and mutism and no real loss of consciousness. *Coma* is total loss of consciousness from which the patient cannot be roused by ordinary stimuli.

The level and quality of consciousness vary even in normal states. In pathological states they vary very widely. Alterations of sensorium are usually indicative of organic pathology.

Disturbances of Biological Functions

Sleep disturbances: These are very common complaints in psychiatry. Sleep is disturbed in several ways, in its pattern, quality and duration. *Insomnia* is lack of sleep which may be total or partial. Total insomnia occurs in several conditions, like mania. Inability to fall asleep (initial insomnia) occurs in anxiety as against late insomnia or waking up early which usually accompanies depression. Sleep—wake pattern is, disturbed in many organic conditions—like delirium or dementia. Sleep may be non-refreshing or inadequate or characterized by frequent waking up or nightmares. In contrast, sleep may be unduly prolonged (*hypersomnia*) or characterized by undue drowsiness in the day time (*somnolence*).

Appetite: *Appetite* is reduced in several psychiatric conditions like anxiety and depression and increased in others like mania. *Pica* refers to eating unedible items like soil, paper, hair, etc. and is a perverted form of appetite. Polydipsia is excessive drinking of water.

Sexual desire: *Sexual desire* is also altered in several psychiatric conditions. It may be increased or decreased. Loss of libido, erectile dysfunctions, ejaculatory disturbances and pain characterize psychosexual disorders.

3

Schizophrenia

Schizophrenia is a heterogeneous group of psychotic disorders and not a single disease entity as is generally believed. The term was introduced by Bleuler to replace its earlier name "dementia praecox" used by Kraeplin. The disease, however, had been recognized in very ancient times as can be seen from the contemporary writings of such periods. In India, for example, medical texts like Charaka Samhita, compiled by Charaka carry clinical descriptions similar to those of present day schizophrenia.

INCIDENCE

Even though schizophrenia may occur in people of any age, it particularly affects adolescents and young adults. The life time risk to develop the illness is about 1% with an incidence between 10 and 15 per 10,000 per year. It affects people of all races and culture, both urban and rural and of both sexes.

Box 3.1: Kraepelin and Dementia Praecox
Emil Kraepelin (1856–1926) German Psychiatrist and Professor of Psychiatry at the university of Munich developed a system of classification of mental illnesses depending on their symptoms and long-term course. He divided the different forms of insanity into two groups. One had an episodic course with relapses and remission but with full recovery after each relapse. This he named manic depressive insanity. The other was a progressive and continuous illness. Starting at adolescence ("praecox") it had a steady down hill course ultimately leading to dementia or total deterioration. This he called dementia praecox. As is now known the illness starts outside adolescence period and does not always lead to dementia. Therefore, the term dementia praecox has only a historic importance.

Box 3.2: Bleuler (1857–1939)

Eugen Bleuler, Swiss Psychiatrist and Director of the Zurich Mental Hospital coined the term schizophrenia in 1911. The word literally means "splitting of mental functions". Bleuler believed that there are two sets of symptoms in schizophrenia — the fundamental symptoms and accessory symptoms. Fundamental symptoms are necessary for a diagnosis of schizophrenia and consist of Autism (extreme withdrawal from reality to phantasy), Ambivalence (simultaneous occurrence of contradictory feelings or ideas), Affective blunting or incongruence and disturbances of association (loss of association in thinking) all these together are known as the four A's of Bleuler. Accessory symptoms are secondary and are of less importance for the diagnosis. Hallucinations, delusions, catatonic symptoms, etc. constitute this group.

TYPES

Clinically there are four main types of the illness. They are:

1. Paranoid schizophrenia
2. Hebephrenic schizophrenia
3. Catatonic schizophrenia and
4. Simple schizophrenia

CLINICAL FEATURES

The clinical features vary depending on the type of schizo-phrenia. They also vary depending on the duration of symptoms, that is the clinical features of an "acute" disorder are different from those of a "chronic" one. Symptoms vary depending on the culture and social background of the patient and even in the same patient they may vary from time to time.

PARANOID SCHIZOPHRENIA

Paranoid (Gr. Para = beside + noeo = to think) schizophrenia is the commonest type and has a later age of onset, often mid twenties or thirties. The characteristic symptoms are delusions which are bizarre and illogical and often expanding, that is, they involve more number of people and situations and becomes stronger over the course of time. Persecutory delusions are the most frequent, though all types of delusions may be present. The patient is distrustful and suspicious of people around, including his own family members. He thinks that he is the point of reference in their conversation. He "discovers" and believes that there are sinister plans in their dealings with him, that they plan to poison or kill him or inflict bodily injuries; or that electrical gadgets are implanted on his body or cameras are set up to spy on him. The patient believes that he is being influenced by cosmic rays or witchcraft or through telepathy. He interprets other people's actions in this light, as for example, when people spit he believes they are spitting at him to show their contempt; when they smile he believes they are laughing at him. Somebody coughing is interpreted as a signal directed at him. Along with delusions the patient may have various types of vivid hallucinations — most frequently the auditory ones. He hears God's voice addressing him or hears threatening voices of his persecutors or voices commanding him to carry out a particular task. The patient's behavior becomes centred on and determined by these delusions and hallucinations so that often he may act on them like breaking up things or attacking people who he believes are his persecutors. In delusions of grandeur he may consider himself as a great leader, inventor or scientist. The patient's other mental functions may be well intact. Though guarded and suspicious he appears alert about his surroundings and organized in his dealings.

Box 3.3: Charaka Samhita

Charaka Cira 100 AD

Charaka Samhita literally meaning the compendium of Charaka is a monumental text of Ayurveda—the ancient system of Indian Medicine. Many forms of insanity were recognized and described. One description goes like this. "Dirty and loathsome he sits secluded or wanders about purposelessly, like a cart without a driver. He talks incoherently, smiles inappropriately, laughs, dances and sings; moves his eyebrows, shoulders, arms and legs purposelessly; sees light, flames of fire, lightning, etc. even though they are not present; adorns himself with rags and things which are dirty and discarded by others; eats gluttonously food which is stale and uneatable." Though supernatural forces were attributed as causative in some types of illnesses Charaka maintained that "neither Gods nor Gandharvas nor Goblins nor Demons torment the mind of man who is not tormented itself by his bad deeds". Mental diseases were classified into different types depending on the clinical picture.

CASE 1

Mrs. GK, a 32-year-old school teacher and mother of two children came to the hospital complaining that she was constantly harassed by her neighbour, an elderly lady, a spinster working as a bank manager in the city. She had moved to the patient's neighbourhood some months before, shortly after which, according to the patient, the harassment started. On one occasion, she visited the patient in her house and while returning "purposefully" left her handbag behind. The patient's husband who also taught in the same school had to take the handbag to its owner. Mrs. GK doubted whether it was a plan to "snatch" her husband from her and later become convinced that it was. She warned her husband not to have any dealings with their neighbour in future. He was prevented from going to the side of that house and from opening windows facing it. She became negligent of her household work and spent her time wandering through the house from one room to another watching her neighbour. She was frequently seen looking at the house standing behind closed curtains. She stopped going to the school and did not permit her husband to leave her premises.

A month after her neighbour's arrival Mrs. GK started hearing voices, telling obscene things and in between calling her "pisachu" (meaning demoness) Mrs. GK identified the voices as her neighbour's. She reported that her neighbour was spying on her peeping into their bedroom with a "telescope like thing" fitted with infrared lenses so that she could see the patient and her husband even in darkness. Her sleep was undisturbed in the beginning but later it started suffering. She said she was woken up by tapping sounds made on the bed room door from outside by the neighbour beckoning her husband when Mrs. GK was asleep.

Patients write endless letters to authorities of law requesting them to act against the tormentors. They might threaten the tormenters directly or even carry out violent acts in offence or defence. Sometimes patients flee from the offending premises in order to get away from their persecutors only to find that they are present in their new dwelling place also. Patients approach the hospital pleading to save them from the offending "radiation or currents" to which they are constantly subjected to or to take away the "electrical" gadgets implanted in their body by the enemies.

HEBEPHRENIA

Hebephrenia (Gr: *Hebe* = puberty + *phren* = the mind) has an early onset of symptoms usually manifesting around adolescence. Among schizophrenias hebephrenia causes the greatest disintegration of personality and the patient rapidly regresses to a childish state with a no-return to normalcy.

The characteristic symptoms are marked incoherence of speech, bizarreness of behavior and silly, incongruous and shallow affect. Because of the incoherence it is difficult to understand the patient's speech dominated by neologisms and abnormalities of thoughts. One patient when asked to write about his life's ambitions wrote the following lines (Fig. 3.1).

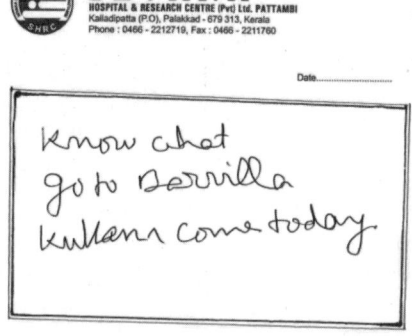

Fig. 3.1: Writing by a hebephernic patient: as can be seen the passage in incoherent and incomprehensible

The bizarreness of behavior is seen in the mannerisms of his speech and activity, facial grimaces, meaningless gestures, etc. Many indulge in baby talk and silly giggling. Making faces, lip pouting and purposeless hyperactivity are common. One patient indulged in walking about in tiptoe the whole day. When asked about this the patient replied that she was "following the order of creation and not even Darwin could change it". Many patients posture in front of the mirror gazing at it for hours together. Patients may indulge in obscene behavior both in talk and activity without any sense of shame or social inhibition. They may play with urine and fecal matter, smearing it over their body or on the floor and walls. The patient's affect is shallow and often incongruent with rapid shifts from weeping to laughing with no appropriate reason. There are violent outbursts of anger which may rapidly pass off again with no adequate cause.

Along with the above symptoms hebephrenic patients will have various types of hallucinations and delusions. Visual and auditory hallucinations are most common and are vivid and fantastic with symbolic interpretations. The contents may change radically from one moment to another. Thus, while the voices make derogatory remarks about the patient at one instant it may change suddenly and "make him laugh" at another. Delusions are of a sexual, religious, grandiose or persecutory nature.

CASE 2

14-year-old Nisha (not the real name), student of 8th std. in a reputed school in the city was expelled from the school for her "unruly behavior and for not obeying her teachers in spite of several warnings". She had been a bright student till a year prior to this, a regular topper in the class who excelled in games and sports also. The change in behavior was noted after a short excursion in which all the students of her class participated. A few days after this, Nisha announced in the open class that she was pregnant as she was hugged by Prince, one of her classmates during the journey. When Nisha told this to her parents they contacted the Principal of the school and discovered that there was nobody in that name in her class. She became inattentive in the class and her performance at school started deteriorating. While in class she giggled without any reason, and appeared self preoccupied, muttering and smiling to self, unmindful of others and time. She remained in her seat after the school hours till she was "woken up" and sent home. When questions were asked in the class she rambled unintelligibly. She became easily irritated and tore the pages of her books or flung the book at others including the teacher. On and off she complained of splitting headaches and was taken by her parents to a neurologist where all investigations gave negative results. At this stage she was expelled from the school.

When seen in psychiatry Nisha said that she was an Arab Queen. She complained of severe headache caused by snakes dwelling inside her head, and constantly striking from inside. At the next moment she laughed aloud and said she was pregnant and would give birth to a snake. Her talk was incoherent and her affect rapidly shifted from gaiety to anger and sorrow. She had clear auditory hallucinations in which Prince spoke to her of their future plans. She had other hallucinations as well. In one she saw "infernal" men in "sky deep blue colour" who asked her to "cut them through" and in another saw insects which were "big as cats " and had heads at both ends. With medicines she improved marginally and was permitted to continue her studies on a trial basis. But in the school her symptoms became worse and studies had to be discontinued.

CATATONIC SCHIZOPHRENIA

The characteristic features of the catatonic (Gr. *Katatonos* = stretching down) type are motor disturbances manifested as stupor, excitement and other abnormalities.

In stupor the patient remains motionless maintaining the same fixed posture for hours together if not disturbed. Various postures are assumed (Fig. 3.2) which are sometimes difficult to break. The patient is mute and retains saliva in mouth which may escape and drool down from the mouth. There is no bladder or bowel control. Even painful stimuli may not elicit any response in a stuporous patient. However on "waking up" the patient is aware of all happenings while in stupor and can relate them in detail.

In excitement the patient shows extreme psychomotor agitation talking and shouting incoherently and running about purposelessly. He may be impulsive and may attack people and destroy things.

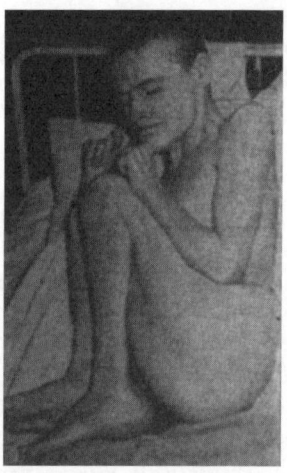

Fig. 3.2: Posture maintained by a patient suffering from schizophrenia. Though uncomfortable the pose is held with no change for very long period of time

Impulsivity and frenzy make the catatonic patients dangerous to himself and others.

Other abnormalities of motor behavior include negativism, ambivalence, waxy flexibility and the various stereotypes like echolalia and echopraxia described in an earlier chapter on signs and symptoms.

Along with the motor disturbances, the patient will have other psychotic symptoms like hallucinations, delusions and mood disturbances. Talk may be incoherent. Like other schizophrenics catatonics also neglect self care and unless attended to become emaciated due to starvation.

CASE 3

An 18-year-old male was admitted with a week long history of social aloofness, not taking food and sleeplessness. To start with some two weeks earlier he stopped talking spontaneously and answered to questions only when they were repeated several times. Even this he stopped a couple of days later and became totally mute prior to coming to the hospital. When spoken to he would look at the speaker blankly without replying. He withdrew to his room and was seen sitting on his bed and gazing into space. At mealtime he sat in front of the plate for a long time and took a few morsels of food. Two days prior to his admission he stopped taking food.

After admission his condition deteriorated and he became stuporous and totally mute. He lay immobile on his cot without changing position for hours together with eyes open gazing at the walls. The attending nurse had to change his position frequently. He was tube fed and catheterized.

On recovery a few weeks later he was able to recall all events and said some outside force was directing his actions. He told that countless voices were simultaneously ordering him what to do and thoughts were racing past through his mind in rapid succession.

SIMPLE SCHIZOPHRENIA

Compared to the other types, simple schizophrenia, does not have any dramatic symptomatology. Lack of florid clinical features characterize this disorder. Starting insidiously at an early age it progresses steadily so that at the end of a few years the patient is visibly converted to the status of a living dummy, with no initiative or interest in the world around him or even in himself. He avoids all social contacts and stops caring for his family or friends. He has no interest in working and if prodded to work does it in a slovenly fashion. Sluggish and apathetic he pulls on with no plans for the future nor ambition, spending most of his time inside his room. Pleading or coaxing or criticizing from the well meaning friends and family members have no effect and he continues to be obstinate and evasive leading a dependent and parasitic life. There are no delusions nor hallucinations and speech through scanty is coherent.

CASE 4

GX, a 30-year-old male was brought to the hospital by his parents for his repeated acts of violence at home. The latest incident occurred that day morning when he pushed his mother down the stairs causing fracture of her right thighbone. Violence was restricted to parents in response to trifling matters like asking him to take food or attend work. About half a dozen episodes had occurred within a period of 3 years but none as serious as the present one.

GX is a graduate and was a student of law some eleven years before. He stopped studies after deciding not to appear for the final examination of the professional course. In school, he was an average student and was regular in attending classes. In college, his performance became poor and he managed to get through BA with the minimum marks needed for a pass. His father, a practicing lawyer got him a seat in the law college. GX was irregular in attending classes in the law college. He skipped classes telling he was unwell and complained of tiredness. The family doctor could not identify any illness even on repeated examinations. He skipped several sessional examinations telling that he had not prepared that portion. In the final year he announced that law was not the profession for him and decided not to write the final examination. He returned home without informing anybody, not even the few friends which he had in the college.

At home he spent most of his time lying on bed gazing at the ceiling. He took food alone, after all others left the table. He stayed awake most of the night and slept till noon. Was not interested in watching TV or reading newspapers. Relented people visiting him. He wore the same dress for days together and did not wash or shave for several days. He secluded more and more to the confines of his room, coming out only to take food. Even the food habits were erratic. All attempts to take him to a psychiatrist failed as he physically resisted them.

His uncle tried to engage him in work in a printing press which he owned but did not succeed. GX seldom went to the press and on reaching there left immediately telling he would start work the next day. When his father coaxed him to do any work he flared up and retreated to his room. On a few occasions he bit his father when provoked to move out of the room. He pushed his mother that day for asking him to wash and dress.

At the clinic GX was cooperative and casual as if nothing significant had happened. He talked clearly and relevantly. All his mental functions were normal. When asked why he pushed his mother he replied that she was meddling in his personal matters and that he lost temper "this once" just as anybody else.

SCHIZOPHRENIA LIKE DISORDERS

There are several conditions which resemble schizophrenia but do not fulfill all its diagnostic criteria. They are mainly four:

1. Those which have an acute onset and are short lived, resolving within a few days or weeks. These are the acute and transient psychotic disorders.

2. Those which have prominent affective (elation or depression) coloring and are called schizoaffective disorders.

3. Those which resemble schizophrenia but lack all its criteria, runs a chronic course and may at a later stage evolve as schizophrenia proper. These are the schizotypal disorders.

4. The fourth group is a heterogeneous one in which persistent, long standing delusions are the only or the most prominent features. These are called as persistent delusional disorders and are dealt in the next chapter.

Box 3.4: First Rank Symptoms of Schizophrenia

Kurt Schneider (1887–1967) German psychiatrist identified a group of symptoms which are diagnostic of schizophrenia. He called them "symptoms of first rank" which when present a diagnosis of schizophrenia can be made with certainly as they are not found in other disorders. They are

1. *Thought echo*: Hearing one's own thoughts spoken aloud.
2. *Third person hallucinations* where voices make remarks about the patient in third person.
3. *Hallucinations in the form of commentary*: Voices speaking usually in the form of a running commentary about the patient's thought and actions.
4. *Thought withdrawal*: Thoughts taken away from the mind.
5. *Thought insertion*: Other people's thoughts inserted into his mind.
6. *Thought broadcast*: One's thoughts accessible to others who make them public.
7. *Passivity feelings*: Patient reports that his thoughts, feelings and actions are not his own but are made and controlled by an external agency.
8. *Delusional perception*: Patient gets sudden revelations and "discovers" "inner meanings" in everyday perception.

Symptoms like perplexity, emotional blunting, delusions and hallucinations were called by Schneider as "second rank symptoms".

Box 3.5: Positive and Negative Symptoms

During its course schizophrenia exhibits both "positive" and "negative" symptoms. The former are those which are seen during active phase of the illness with which they coincide. The symptoms are florid and makes the illness obvious. When this passes off either naturally or as a result of treatment the patient recovers either fully which is rare or to a great extent. In the latter case, when recovery is not complete it leaves back some residual symptoms, the pockmarks of a previous active illness. These are the negative symptoms.

Positive symptoms	*Negative symptoms*
Hallucinations	Affective blunting
Delusions	Apathy
Catatonic symptoms	Psychomotor slowing and underactivity
Thought disturbances	Lack of initiative and will
Anomalies of mood	Poverty of thinking
	Social withdrawal
	Anhedonia (lack of pleasure)

In general, positive symptoms are the characteristic of an acute illness or acute exacerbation and negative symptoms characteristic of a chronic illness.

ETIOLOGY

Biological, psychological and sociological factors are believed to underlie causation of the illness. Biological and psychological factors are of prime importance and determine the predisposition for the illness. Social factors precipitate an episode. The relative importance and interplay of factors vary from patient to patient.

Biological Factors

 i. **Heredity:** Family studies and studies on twins indicate that heredity is an important factor. Monozygotic (identical) twins are 3 times more affected than dizygotic (fraternal) twins. Mode of inheritance is not known. Some studies support the hypothesis that schizophrenia results from a cumulative effect of multiple genes while other studies support a single gene effect. Some forms of schizophrenia are believed to have no genetic influence.

 ii. **Biochemical anomalies:** Various biochemical anomalies, are attributed as causative, as dopamine hyperactivity, increased norepinephine activity and serotonin anomalies (excess or deficiency).

 iii. **Cerebral factors:** Brain studies show cortical atrophy and ventricular dilatation in about one third of schizophrenic patients. This is attributed to the longstanding effects of infection of discrete parts of the brain by slow neurotropic viruses.

Psychological Factors

Persons with certain types of personality (as for example, schizoid personality) characterized by social aloofness and withdrawal, "cold" and friendless individuals are more; prone to have the illness in later life.

Sociological Factors

Pathological family patterns have been pointed out as causative factors. One pathological pattern is where the parental roles are reversed ("He-wife" and "She-husband"). Broken homes, unstable marital relationships, eccentric child rearing practices and indulgence of parents in undercutting each other are other forms anomalous family environment.

Migration and other radical changes in life style are other sociological factors which may precipitate the illness.

DIAGNOSIS

The diagnosis of schizophrenia should be made only after longitudinal and cross sectional studies through history and mental status examination respectively. "Straight" and typical cases do not offer any difficulty. Table 3.1 lists the ICD-10 criteria for the diagnosis of schizophrenia.

According to the International Classification one or more clear cut symptoms from list A and/or two or more from list B should be present for most of the time during a period of one month or more for diagnosing schizophrenia.

Box 3.6: Model Psychosis

Psychosis like states can be artificially induced by administration of hallucinogenic drugs or by sensory deprivation. The Swiss chemist, Hofmann who synthesized LSD in 1938 self administered it to observe its effects (which he called "harrowing"). When the results of these self trials were published, it stimulated latter researchers to use similar psychotomimetic agents (like Mescakine, LSD, etc.) to study the aetiology of schizophrenia. However, it was soon found out model psychoses produced by drugs were different from schizophrenia and were akin to organic psychoses producing delirious states in high doses. Another way to produce model psychoses is by sensory deprivation, that is, by deliberately cutting out all sensory inputs (visual, auditory, tactile, etc.) of the individual.

In one design the subjects wearing special head masks for breathing were immersed in a cubicle filled with tepid water. Eyes were covered with goggles and ears with sponge pads, the arms were splintered and extremities wrapped. After some time the subjects craved for stimulation, became restless and reported psychotic symptoms like hallucinations and delusions. The clinical picture in sensory deprivation resembles schizophrenia more than in drug induced psychotic states.

Table 3.1: Criteria for diagnosis of schizophrenia

List A	List B
a. Thought disturbance (echo, inserton, withdrawal, broadcasting)	a. Persistent hallucinations of any modality
b. Delusions (control, passivity, delusional perception)	b. Incoherent speech, irrelevant talk, thought block, neologism
c. Persistent delusions which are culturally inappropriate or which are impossible (like being able to control weather)	c. Catatonic symptoms
d. Hallucinations in third person, running commentary, or hallucinations coming from different parts of body	d. Negative symptoms of any type, not drug induced or part of other illness (e.g. depression)
	e. Overall deterioration of personality

When all the clinical features have not fully developed and in atypical presentations schizophrenia is to be differentiated from many other conditions.

DIFFERENTIAL DIAGNOSIS

i. **Affective disorders:** Affective disorders may present with or without psychotic features. In either mood disturbance is the primary symptom. Psychotic symptoms appear later and usually do not persist for long. Family history, premorbid personality, age of onset (affective disorders usually have a later age of onset) and response to treatment are helpful clues. First rank symptoms are absent.

ii. **Drug induced psychosis:** Alcohol, LSD, cannabis, amphetamine, steroids, etc. can induce psychosis. Careful history provides clues. Many drugs have their characteristic symptoms (e.g. tactile hallucinations in cocaine, visual ones in LSD) cognitive disturbances affecting sensorium, are usually present in many of them.

iii. **Acute and transitional disorders:** History, and course of the illness are differentiating points.

iv. **Neurological disorders:** Infections (as Herpes encephalitis, HIV, etc.) seizure disorders (particularly temporal lobe epilepsy), tumors (particularly those of frontal and temporal regions), degenerative conditions (e.g. Huntington's chorea), etc. produce psychotic symptoms. History, neurological examination and investigations help diagnosis.

v. **Severe obsessive compulsive disorder:** An obsessional thought resembles a delusion because of its magical nature. But in obsessional disorders the patient resists them and understands them as foreign ("ego alien" whereas in schizophrenia the patient accepts them as true and without resistance ("ego syntonic").

vi. **Personality disorders:** Paranoid, schizoid, dissocial and emotionally unstable personality disorders are to be differentiated from schizophrenia. Psychotic symptoms are absent in personality disorders.

vii. **Schizoaffective disorders:** Definite symptoms of schizophrenia and affective symptoms should be present simultaneously and prominently in schizoaffective disorders.

viii. **Delusional disorders:** Delusions in delusional disorders are non bizarre and logical. Hallucinations are usually absent. There is no deterioration of personality.

ix. **Medical conditions:** Some medical conditions (particularly endocrine disorders like Cushing's syndrome (hyperadrenalism) and myxoedema (hypothyroidism) have mood changes and psychotic symptoms as delusions. Relevant investigations are helpful.

x. **Mental retardation:** Sometimes resembles simple schizophrenia. But in mental retardation the poor level of functioning is stable and constant. There is no progressive deterioration.

xi. **Malingering:** Cases have been reported where malingerers were successful in initiating schizophrenic symptoms. Careful history repeated to discover any underlying secondary gain and indirect observation without patient's knowledge will clear the issue.

Box 3.7: Famous People with Schizophrenia

Schizophrenia does not respect geographical or man made boundaries. Or other differences like sex, race, culture, caste and creed. It can afflict any human being from the most famous to the most ignoramus. One name belonging to the first group is that of Mary Todd Lincoln, wife of America's 15th president, Abraham Lincoln. Following death of her 11-year-old son she had a psychotic break down. She was later diagnosed to be suffering from schizophrenia. John Nash, Nobel Laurette (economics, 1994) and a great mathematician, inventor of the Nash Equilibria was once diagnosed to have paranoid schizophrenia. A Hollywood film, "a beautiful mind" is based on his mathematical genius and how he struggled with his illness. Another name in the list is that of Jack Kerouac, an American novelist, poet, artist and writer. Jim Gordon, a grammy award winning musician killed his mother acting on hallucinatory voices. Joe Meek was a famous English record producer who was diagnosed to be suffering from schizophrenia. During his life time he was preoccupied with the occult, paranormal and after death happenings and often set up sound recorders in graves to pick up voices coming from the dead. Vaclav Nijinsky was a gifted male dancer from polland who had schizophrenia. The illness affected his career. He was taken to Switzerland where he was treated by Eugene Bleuler. Among those with schizophrenia are singers, artists and painters, poets, writers, sportsman and doctors including psychiatrists.

MANAGEMENT

Patients who pose management problems and those who are at risk for themselves and other people should be hospitalized. For others treatment on an outpatient basis can be tried with regular periodical reviews. Medication should be supervised and should be continued for several weeks or months depending on the clinical condition. Many patients need a maintenance dose of medication for several years to reduce relapses.

Treatments fall under two categories:
1. Somatic or physical methods
2. Psychosocial methods.

SOMATIC METHODS

These include drugs and electoconvulsive therapy.

    i. **Drugs:** Several antipsychotic drugs are currently available which are dealt in Chapter 12. Combination of drugs may be needed to avoid adverse reactions of a single drug given in a heavy dose. Parenteral depot forms are available which considerably reduce the frequency of administration — to once a week or month. Liquid preparations and the recently introduced dispersible tablets help administration without patient's awareness that he is on medication, if this can be suitably manned. Concurrent use of medicines apart from antipsychotics may be necessary — like antitremor agents to combat extrapyramidal side effects or hypnotics to induce sleep whenever needed.

ii. **Electroconvulsive therapy:** ECT is helpful in a small percentage of patients, particularly when they are stuporous and when there are positive symptoms.

PSYCHOSOCIAL METHODS

These include individual, group and family therapy sessions. Occupational therapy is helpful when the acute symptoms are controlled and the patient is more manageable.

Half way homes and day care centers provide after care facilities and are part of rehabilitation.

COURSE AND PROGNOSIS

Many patients have residual symptoms in spite of timely treatment and partial recovery. The long-term course of the illness varies from patient-to-patient and may take one of the several forms as shown in Fig. 3.3.

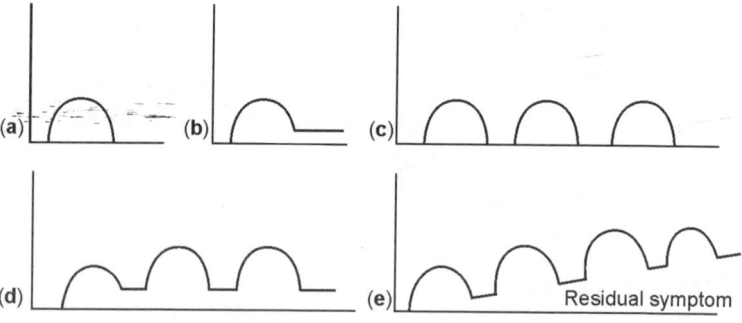

Fig. 3.3: Outcome of schizophrenia (a) single episode with full recovery, (b) single episode with incomplete remission, (c) multiple episode with total recovery, (d) multiple episode with stable deficit, (e) multiple episode with progressive deficit

Prognosis is better in paranoid and catatonic types of schizophrenia. Indicators of good prognosis are tabulated in Table 3.2.

Table 3.2: Predictors of good outcome
1. Acute onset and short duration of symptoms (less than 3 months)
2. Older age at onset
3. Presence of stressful events or situation as precipitating factors
4. Absence of previous psychiatric history
5. Absence of family history of schizophrenia
6. Presence of depressive illness in the family
7. Stable premorbid personality with no schizoid traits
8. Presence of perplexity or confusional symptoms
9. Preservation of affect
10. Good supportive systems in the family and community

4

Delusional Disorders

Delusional disorders, like schizophrenia are a group of heterogeneous conditions where paranoid symptoms are the most conspicuous feature. There is no associated illness which could account for their occurrence. Their presence, persistence and impact on behavior are the factors which lead the patient for a consultation. The delusion may be a single one or there may be a number of them involving a set of related people and situations.

In medical practice, paranoid symptoms appear in a variety of clinical conditions. The word "paranoid", like anxiety or depression is a descriptive term, not a diagnostic one. In the setting of a personality disorder paranoid symptoms appear as excessive self reference and tendency to attribute malevolent motives in the actions of others. They can occur in association with several primary psychiatric conditions like schizophrenia, mood disorder and substance abuse and in many medical conditions, as for example epilepsy and myxedema. Either of them, however, does not qualify as a delusional disorder. In personality disorder they are not true delusions but are only paranoid ideas and in the latter they are secondary to an already existing primary illness.

INCIDENCE

Little is known about the true incidence and prevalence of the disorder. They were once considered uncommon and rare. Some studies indicate that the incidence is 1–3 cases per 10,000 persons per annum with prevalence between 0.03 and 0.07%. Women are affected more and the age of onset is late thirties or forties or later.

CLINICAL SUBTYPES

Five subtypes of delusional disorders are recognized according to one classification system.

1. Persecutory type
2. Grandiose type
3. Jealous type
4. Erotomanic type
5. Somatic type

CLINICAL FEATURES

In general, the clinical features are the presence of delusions, the associated mood changes and their impact on the patient's work and behavior. There are no "cognitive" (higher mental function) disturbances.

Delusions

Though the content differs the delusions in all the subtypes have some common characteristics.

a. **Dominance:** Delusions are the most conspicuous features and they dominate the clinical picture.

b. **Nonbizarreness:** Unlike in schizophrenia delusions are logical and comprehensible and are conceivable in ordinary life situations, for example, a delusion that he is spied upon by his neighbour. Compare this with the bizarre delusion of a schizophrenic, as for example, aliens from another planet are controlling his actions through a remote mechanism.

c. **Encapsulation:** Delusions are isolated and they do not pervade other mental functions of the patient or disturb the integrity of his functioning.

d. **Persistence:** Delusions persist over a long period of time and may not totally disappear.

e. **Systematization:** A single delusion may become elaborated and well systematized by incorporating several secondary delusions related to the original theme. Over a course of time the patient spins a complicated net work of delusions.

Mood

The mood is appropriate to the contents of the delusion. There is no incongruity.

Hallucinations

Hallucinations are usually absent. If present they are not prominent. However in the somatic type patient may have tactile hallucinations — like worms crawling under the skin, etc.

Negative symptoms

Unlike in schizophrenia negative symptoms are nil or minimal in delusional disorders. There is no appreciable personality deterioration.

PERSECUTORY TYPE

Here the theme of the delusion is persecutory. The patient believes that he is the centre of a plot in which people around (or a selected gang of people) are working against him. They conspire to harass, dislodge, poison or kill him with an ulterior motive like taking away his property or position. The patient may complain to the police or write letters to the authorities requesting protection from enemies. He may even resort to violence against his supposed persecutors.

Box 4.1
Mozart, the great composer had delusions that he was being poisoned. The French philosopher Jean Jaeques Rosseau had marked paranoid ideas and believed that secret enemies from England and France sent by the King and priests were plotting to kill him through poisoned vegetables. He alleged his stomach upsets to poisoning. On one occasion he "discovered" such a plot while he was in his hotel and ran away in panic leaving all his belongings in the hotel room. He implored to be put in a prison where he thought he would be safe from his persecutors. He wrote a letter to God pleading to save him from enemies and went to place the letter on the altar of Notre-dame Cathedral at Paris. He could not take it to the altar and became convinced that God also was against him.

Navaz, a 37-year clerk who was working in a finance company applied for a personal loan which was turned down by the management. Navaz attributed this to his low social status as he belonged to a minority community and to the weak recommendation made in this regard by his "upper class" manager. Navaz confided this to his colleague with whom he shared his room in town. A week later while in office Navaz saw a police jeep alight in front of the finance company and two policemen enter the manager's cabin. After a short while Navaz was summoned and was asked to bring a particular file to the office. Navaz became afraid and deduced that the manager knew everything which he had confided to his friend the other day. He thought his friend acted as a stoolpigeon and the manager had called the police to lodge a complaint against Navaz for "spreading scandals against the company". He believed his being called to the office was a ploy to show his identity to the police. He took leave for the rest of the day and immediately shifted his residence to another part of the town without even telling his friend. He did not go out fearing the police, did not take his evening meals and did not sleep in the night. He rang up to his house the next day to enquire whether any police officer had come there asking for him. He told his wife that the manager had sacked him and wanted to get rid of him with the help of police. He was brought home and then to the hospital.

Navaz was convinced that there was a secret gang working against him in the office headed by his manager. He thought that he was being constantly watched since the moment he applied for the loan by his own colleagues who had tipped his former room mate "to find out all his secrets". He knew that his phone was "being tapped by the manager and was denied access to any incoming calls" as he did not receive any calls from outside during this period. The policemen had come to the premises to pressurize him to resign and would have taken him into custody but for his "lucky escape in the niche of time".

At the end of two weeks on medicines there was only marginal improvement of his symptoms. A month later he resigned his job. He was at that time as convinced as he was at the time of starting the treatment and believed that he was being harassed because of his minority status. Navaz had at no time any evidence of hallucinations or other perceptual disturbances.

Box 4.2: Don Quixote

Who has not read the adventures of Don Quixote, Cervantes' comic satire against the chivalric romances? Don Quixote who is bemused by reading stories of chivalry decides to be a knight himself and sets out on his old horse Rosimante seeking new adventures. He is accompanied by Sancho Panza, a poor farmer from the village, as his Squire. Don Quixote was convinced that he had a great mission to fulfil that is to defend the oppressed and to right injustice which would bring fame and honour to him. He wanted stories of his famous deeds and bravery to be read by all people. He fought against his perceived enemies and giants which however, turned out to be wind mills and wine skins. On another occasion he saw two flocks of sheep which he took as two groups of rival armies attacking each other and went to the rescue of the weaker group. The delusional conviction that he is the chosen one to pursue a particular mission and the unquestioned belief that he has the skill and energy to fulfill it are the clinical features of the grandiose type of delusional disorders.

CASE 2

GK, a 60-year-old retired teacher hailing from a middle class family constantly remarked of his huge industrial complex in aneighbouring state "managed by his cousins for convenience sake". The complex along with an adjacent 60 acre estate and bungalow, GK believed, was bequeathed to him by its one time owner, to be expertly managed by him personally after the former's death, as his children were inept and inefficient. For twenty years after the owner's death, GK would go to the estate once a month unfailingly meet the manager and ask him whether everything was Ok in the estate. He insisted and left word with the manager that any unruly happening in the estate should be reported to him personally. The manager and the estate's rightful owners kept GK in good humour each time he visited them as he was one of their cousins though he had no legal right to any of the possessions.

GK was an excellent teacher and recipient of an award instituted by the State Govt, for being the best teacher of the year. He was a dear both to his students and family members.

GRANDIOSE TYPE

In the grandiose type the patients are convinced about their possession of special powers or talents which others have not yet recognized. They may believe that they belong to the "chosen few" to lead the masses or to contribute substantially to the betterment of mankind. Legacy to huge assets and property or their intellectual achievements are their constant ruminations even though there is no factual basis for any such claims.

JEALOUS TYPE

The central theme in this type is a delusion of infidelity. The husband or wife believes that his or her partner is unfaithful and carries on extramarital relationships in secret. The proofs on which the allegations are based are often tangential or are incorrect and without adequate support like casual glances at members of the opposite sex, late home comings, stains on clothes, or disarrayed dress. They often coerce confession from their partners many a time at threats of physical harm or even violent acts. Doors are marked with tapes, mirrors adjusted or agencies notified for detective work against the suspected partner.

Box 4.3: Othello Syndrome

The delusional disorder where one's spouse is charged with infidelity is sometimes called as "Othello syndrome" after Othello, immortalized by Shakespeare. Among his two subordinates—Cassio and Iago—the former is appointed by Othello, as the Moorish General or his chief lieutenant. The envious Iago takes revenge by falsely implicating Othello's wife, Desdemona and Cassio in a love affair secretly planting in Cassio's robes, a handkerchief gifted to Desdemona by Othello. The handkerchief is recovered from Cassio's room. Othello, the jealous husband convinced about his wife's infidelity kills her and later kills himself.

CASE 3

HM, a 53-year-old teacher, married for 29 years came with his wife to the hospital allegedly for the latter's treatment. His wife, also a teacher worked in a different school, nearer to their home than the school where the husband taught. According to HM for the past two years his wife had been leaving to school earlier than himself, even though he had to travel a longer distance. Also she returned late, much later than her husband. His wife attributed this to the special classes in the evening. She had to leave early in the morning as she had to take her grand daughter who was studying in the same school.

HM, alleged that his wife was involved with her headmaster or other male teachers and had sexual relations with them while at school. On several occasions HM took leave from his school to check on his wife and visited her school on some pretext or other. At no time he called on his wife but talked to her colleague teachers and enquired whether she had been visiting her headmaster frequently in his office. At no time he had seen her with the headmaster or with any other males but he continued to believe that she was able to foretell his arrival in the school and take precautions against getting caught red-handed. Whenever confronted by HM his wife would tell that she was innocent and that the allegations were untrue.

HM reported that of late his wife started entertaining her lovers even at home while he was asleep, which according to him was the need of the immediate consultation. His proofs were several in number. He was sleeping more than usual, and woke up late in the morning, which he attributed to his wife putting sleeping pills in the evening coffee. She was changing the bed linen more frequently. There were marks of cycle tyres on the ground and one of her colleagues had a bicycle. Wife smelled of tobacco which neither she nor HM was in the habit of using while her colleagues were smokers. On one occasion he picked up the stump of a cigarette which according to him was thrown away after smoking by her paramour. Further his neighbours were smiling at him in a "we-know-all" fashion which made him suspect that his wife had the support of his neighbours also in cheating him. He had brought his wife to the hospital for a "thorough advice" against cheating her husband and against hiding the true facts.

EROTOMANIC TYPE

Compared to other types erotomania is rare and usually involves a woman bearing an unshakeable belief that a particular member of the opposite sex usually in an exalted position is deeply infatuated with her and cannot live without her. She believes that because of his high position he is prevented by others from meeting her and expressing his love directly, and therefore, resorts to oblique ways of communication which she alone can understand. Frequently she writes letters or make phone calls or sends gifts to her lover who may be unsuspecting and unaware of the whole affair. Some patients may even resort to constantly surveile or stalk their "prey". If the male is married she may announce that the marriage is invalid and not genuine. The love is often at an idyllic level and may not aim at sexual pleasure seeking. Due to the repeated advances the patient becomes a nuisance to the exasperated male who might resort to all possible ways including help from police to get rid of the patient with varied success.

SOMATIC TYPE

In the somatic type, the delusion involves one's body functions and sensory experiences. Delusions may take several forms. The patient believes that his body is infested with insects or worms which crawls under the skin and cause itching. Some allege emanation of strange smells and foul odour from their body because of which people avoid them. Other delusions involve their internal organs which are shrinking or rotting inside or their body parts which they believe are misshapen and ugly.

Box 4.4: Folie a Deux (Folie = psychosis; deux = two)

Occasionally delusions are transferred from one individual to another when both of them share the same delusions. This almost always happens in a family setting when the dominant member induces his or her delusions onto the passive, more suggestible partner. Usual partners are: sister and sister, husband and wife or mother and child. Sometimes more than two people are simultaneously affected. The delusions disappear when the partners separate-recovery being faster and better in the recipient than in the inducer.

CASE 4

Mrs. W., a 69-year-old widow was referred by a dermatologist whom the patient had consulted for itching all over her face. She attributed this to the presence of tiny worms in her mouth which were creeping over the skin inside the cheek. Mrs. W. maintained that she could see them. In an attempt to demonstrate their presence she gargled and spat out water on the floor. Patient asserted that the white specks on the foamy water were real worms. No explanations to the contrary changed her convictions.

ETIOLOGY

Etiology of delusional disorder is not clear. Biological, environmental and psychodynamical factors are attributed as causative. Family studies show that there is an increased risk of delusional disorder in the first degree relatives of schizophrenic patients but not vice versa. Structural changes in the brain (cortical atrophy and enlargement of ventricles) similar to schizophrenia are seen in delusional disorders also. Substance abuse, particularly alcohol produces symptoms similar to delusional disorders. Some special conditions like imprisonment, migration and culture alienation produce delusional symptoms. Psychodynamic theories hold that persecutory delusions are the result of unconscious homosexual urges which are denied and projected by the individual.

Box 4.5

Certain special situations are fertile grounds for the development of delusions. In experimental conditions sensory deprivation (mentioned in an earlier chapter) can give rise to paranoid symptoms. People migrating to another country or to another place in the same country where language, conduct and behavior are different experience "culture shock" which can precipitate delusional symptoms till acculturization of the individual occurs. Jail inmates waiting trial, prisoners of war and those in solitary confinement develop psychotic symptoms with mainly persecutory type of delusions (prison psychosis). In a few of them this could be related to use of alcohol and other substances.

DIAGNOSIS

Diagnosis is made by the clinical picture with characteristic predominant delusions, which are nonbizarre, well systematized and encapsulated. Table 4.1 summarises the diagnostic criteria according to the Diagnostic and Statistical Manual of Mental Disorders (DSM-IV)

Table 4.1: Diagnostic criteria for delusional disorders according to DSM–IV

1. Presence of delusions which are non-bizarre and which can happen in real life situations. They are of minimum one month duration
2. Absence of characteristic symptoms of schizophrenia like delusions, hallucinations, incoherent speech, catatonic symptoms, negative symptoms and disorganized behaviour
3. Delusions though they might be systemized, are encapsulated and do not markedly disrupt the patient's normal functioning
4. Mood disturbances are secondary to delusions and of shorter duration
5. Symptoms are not due to a general medical condition or due to substance use
6. Tactile and olfactory hallucinations may be present in the somatic subtype of the delusional disorder

DIFFERENTIAL DIAGNOSIS

1. **Paranoid schizophrenia:** Distinguishing features are the nature of delusions (non-bizarre and encapsulated in delusional disorders), absence of hallucinations, preservation of affect and lack of negative symptoms. Age of onset in delusional disorders is latter than in schizophrenia.

2. **Paranoid personality disorder:** There are no true delusions in personality disorder.

3. **Substance abuse:** Cocaine produces tactile hallucinations. Alcohol and amphetamine precipitate delusional symptoms. History will help. Cognitive disturbances are absent in delusional disorders, but are common in substance abuse.

4. **Mood disorders:** Depressed patients often have paranoid delusions. Grandiose delusions are seen in mania. In mood disorders the delusions are secondary to the altered mood and are short lived. Positive family history and course of the illness with remissions and relapses are other distinguishing features in mood disorders.

5. **General medical conditions:** Paranoid delusions are often present in myxedema. Other conditions include Parkinson's disease, multiple sclerosis, Alzheimer's disease and cerebral tumors.

TREATMENT

In delusional disorders, more than in any other psychiatric disorders an objective evaluation of the history provided by the patient and his symptoms are of paramount importance. This is because delusions are logical and involve everyday life situations. Their delusional nature can often be understood only on careful analysis of the context and information obtained from a reliable informant.

Assessment of the severity of delusions and patient's dangerousness (to himself and others) is also important before deciding the treatment plan. Patients who are dangerous because of their delusions should be hospitalized and the concerned people informed. Patients do not consider themselves ill and in need of any treatment. They will skip medicines unless medicines are given under supervision. Antipsychotics and antidepressants (if needed) are the preferred drugs. In the somatic type of delusional disorders pimozide is the drug of choice. Electroconvulsive therapy is not effective.

COURSE AND PROGNOSIS

Delusional disorders have a chronic course in spite of treatment. Many a time the conditions are refractory to medicines and the delusions persist as strongly as before. Drugs are useful to abbreviate associated agitation and aggression.

In more than half of the patients the symptoms remit and relapse with fairly symptom free intervals in between two relapses. A good percentage of them are symptomatically stable over time. About a half of patients have a chronic unremitting course.

5

Mania and Depression

EMOTIONS AND MOOD

In common language the terms emotion, feeling affect and mood are used interchangeably and almost synonymously. They agree with each other in that all of them refer to the mental state of the organism. However, in actual usage there are subtle differences in meaning between these terms.

Emotion (feeling) is one of the three functions of the mind, the other two being cognition (knowing or thinking) and conation (will). It is a difficult term to define, though less hard to describe. Emotion gives color to life and without it life is dull and colorless—a spread of monotonous grey. Emotion motivates the organism to action. Emotions are numerous—fear, dread, panic, apprehension, rage, fury, distrust, scorn, contempt, dismay, shame, remorse, disgust, grief, pity, delight, ecstasy, etc. being some of them. Their responses on the organism are also manifold and involve, internal organic reactions (like rapid pulse, raised blood pressure, tachypnea, sweating, etc.) overt expressive movements (wide open eyes, clenched fists, etc.) and a conscious roused up subjective feeling (fear, rage, etc.). Emotions are acute turbulent conditions and are usually short lived.

Feeling is the pleasure-pain dimension of emotions. It is the experience as reported by the individual, like sadness, joy, tension, calm, etc.

Affects are discrete, strong, transient emotions and refer to the feeling tone, pleasurable or not, that accompanies an idea. They include the inner feelings and their external manifestations. Affect and emotion are often used interchangeably.

When affect is sustained and not transient it is called mood. It denotes the affective state of a relatively long duration. In analogous terms mood refers to the season whereas affect refers to the prevailing weather. Mood is less intense and less turbulent than the emotional reactions.

Mania and depression are two poles of a spectrum of disorders where affect or mood is primarily disturbed. They are therefore called as mood (or affective) disorders. All other changes, i.e. those of cognition and conation are secondary to the altered mood.

Some characteristic features differentiate mood disorders from other conditions. They are: (i) morbid alterations of mood ranging from unwarranted elation or hilarity to extreme gloom or despondence, (ii) associated changes in thought and behavior which are secondary to the mood changes and which are appropriate or congruent to the mood, (iii) tendency of the disorder to recur with symptom-free intervals in between successive episodes and (iv) relative preservation of the patient's personality which does not deteriorate in spite of recurrent episodes of illness.

CLASSIFICATION

Recurrent cycles of "mania" and "melancholia" in the same persons were recognized by physicians as early as 6th century. But it was Kraepelin who became convinced that all these states only represented manifestations of a single morbid process. He introduced the term "manic depressive psychosis" in 1896 to describe a disorder characterised by episodes of elation and depression with periods of relative normality in between and a favorable outcome. Its subtypes were mania, depression and circular psychosis the latter characterised by alternating periods of mania and depression. In 1962, a different system of grouping was suggested depending on the course of illness:

1. Disorders characterized by episodes of depression and depression alone (unipolar depression).
2. Disorder characterized by episodes of elation and elation alone (unipolar mania).
3. Disorder characterized by both depression and mania (bipolar disorder).

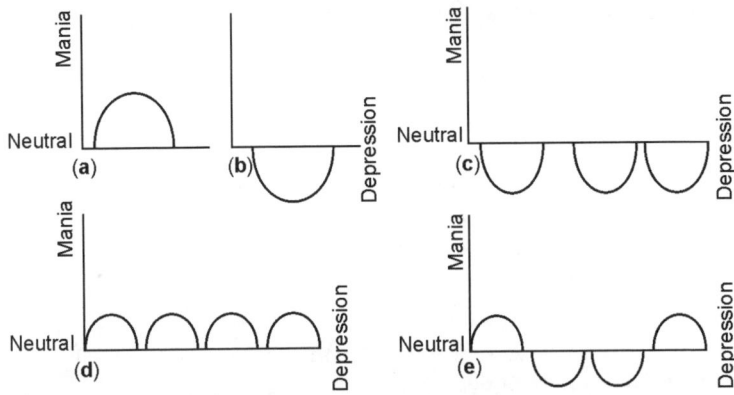

Fig. 5.1: Affective disorder—a schematic diagram (a) single manic episode, (b) single depressive episode, (c) multiple unipolar depressive episodes (recurrent depressive disorder), (d) multiple unipolar manic episodes (called as bipolar disorder), (e) multiple bipolar affective episodes (bipolar affective disorder)

The term unipolar mania is not used as recurrent episodes of mania alone are rare. Moreover, this group resembles the bipolar disorder in all aspects in family history, premorbid personality, age of onset and outcome. Bipolar disorders include unipolar mania also. Unipolar depression is otherwise known as major depressive disorder.

Bipolar I and Bipolar II Disorders

When depression alternates with mania it is sometimes called as Bipolar I disorder. If depression alternates with hypomania (milder form of mania—a state between normal euphoria and mania—(see text)—it is known as Bipolar II disorder.

Classification of affective disorders according to ICD-10 is given in Table 5.1.

EPIDEMIOLOGY

The life time risk for bipolar disorder as well as for mania is about 1 % whereas for unipolar disorders it is 10–15%. Sex ratio (male : female) is 1:1 in bipolar disorder whereas it is 1:2 in unipolar disorders—that is, females are more prone to have a unipolar illness compared to males whereas in bipolar disorders the risk is the same for both sexes. Bipolar disorders affect

Table 5.1: Classification of mood disorders according to ICD-10

A. DEPRESSIVE DISORDER
1. Depressive episode
   Mild
   Moderate
   Severe (with or without psychotic symptoms)
   Atypical
2. Recurrent depressive disorder
   Currently mild
   Currently moderate
   Currently severe (with or without psychotic symptoms)
   Recurrent brief depression

B. MANIC DISORDER
1. Hypomania
2. Mania (with or without psychotic symptoms)

C. BIPOLAR AFFECTIVE DISORDER
1. Currently hypomanic
2. Currently manic (with or without psychotic symptoms)
3. Currently depressed (with or without psychotic symptoms)
4. Current episode mixed

D. PERSISTENT MOOD DISORDER
1. Cyclothymia
2. Dysthymia

younger people, with an average age of onset at 20 whereas in unipolar disorder the average age of onset is 30. Both disorders can, however, affect people at any age. With advancing age depressive episodes become more frequent.

CLINICAL FEATURES

Depression

Depression is the commonest mood disorder which manifests as a single episode or as an episodic or even chronic disorder. In worldwide surveys, it is the fourth most important cause of disability—markedly impairing physical, social, family and work functions of an individual. Symptoms may vary from one person to another or in the same person between two different episodes or at two points of time in the same episode. The symptoms very much overlap with those of anxiety disorders and anxiety may often appear as the only precursor of an oncoming depression. Anxiety may coexist with depression. The symptoms are conveniently grouped under the following heads.

Mood Changes

Mood changes are considered as a necessary condition for diagnosing depression but all patients may not complain of being sad. Instead patients may report of having a "feeling of emptiness", anxiety, anhedonia (lack of pleasure) or "no feelings", and these may be the presenting symptoms.

Cognitive Changes

Negative evaluation of self and the world is characteristic of depression. The depressed person considers himself as the most wretched person on earth, the worst sinner deserving no mercy. The world will be better off without him. He is full of remorse even for minor lapses on his part with morbid guilt feelings. This along with self diffidence adds to his misery and pessimism. Severe hopelessness and helplessness make him think of ending life by committing suicide. Time stands still for him and each moment is perceived as never ending and full of agony.

Biological Functions

Sleep is disturbed. There is difficulty in falling asleep (initial insomnia) and the patient wakes up several hours before his usual waking time (late insomnia). Sleep may be interrupted and marred with nightmares. Appetite is reduced and he may also have anorexia. The patient eats little and may lose weight considerably. All activities are diminished and there is "no energy" to carry on. Interest in sex is usually reduced. Paradoxically some patients have an acceleration of biological energies with an increase in appetite, sleep and sexual feelings.

Behavior Changes

There is profound slowing both in thinking and acting (retardation) or he may be agitated and restlessly moving about.

The patient avoids all forms of social contacts and withdraws from people around the activities which used to interest him earlier are no more pursued. There is no will or concentration in work and even small tasks like washing and dressing are a burden needing great effort. The patient gets tired easily and prefers to lie down all the time neglecting self and personal care.

Box 5.1: Severity of Depression

Depression is graded as mild, moderate and severe depending on the frequency and intensity of symptoms. For this the symptoms are grouped into two: (1) the most typical ones and (2) others. The most typical symptoms are: (a) depressed mood, (b) lack of interest and lack of joy and (c) easy fatigability. Other symptoms of depression are: (a) reduced attention and concentration, (b) self diffidence and loss of self-esteem, (c) ideas of unworthiness and guilt feelings, (d) pessimistic views of future, (e) thoughts or acts of self harm, (f) sleep disturbances and (g) poor appetite. In mild depression a minimum of two symptoms each from the first group and from the second group should be present, which have a minimum two weeks duration and are not very severe. For qualifying depression as moderate there should be a minimum of two typical symptoms and 3–4 other symptoms. The symptoms should be present for two weeks and are more intense. Depression is graded severe when all the three typical symptoms are present along with four or more of the other symptoms. The symptoms are severe enough to disrupt normal work and persist for a period of two weeks. In moderate and severe degrees of depression the duration may be less than two weeks if the symptoms are very severe or if more number of them are present.

Depressive Episode

15–20% of patients suffering from depression do not relapse and have only a single episode. The symptoms persist for several weeks or several months even with medication. Severity of the depression varies from mild to moderate or severe and psychotic symptoms may be present or not.

CASE 1

A 36-year-old company executive working with an oil firm in the gulf countries got himself admitted in the hospital after an attempt of suicide by taking sleeping tablets while in the working place.

He was accompanied by his wife to whom he had been complaining of sleeplessness for the past 3 months, and recurrent wishes "to join his mother" who had died 6 months earlier. The mother, a frail lady ailing from a cardiac illness had not favored her son taking up a job abroad in spite of her other children being around to look after her. Each time the patient left abroad after leave he used to promise her mother that he would to resign and come back permanently after "this once". After mother's death and after the obsequies were performed at home he joined work a few weeks later.

On admission the patient was reluctant to speak except to say that he would kill himself and nobody could stop him. He was full of remorse and occasionally remarked that he was responsible for his mother's death. He said that it was his wife and not himself who prompted the hospital admission — as he believed no medicines could help him. He did not want to continue his job. At night he was sleepless telling that mother was calling him.
With medicines and emotional support he improved and was able to get rid of his guilt feelings. He joined work. Medicines were continued for about six months and were later stopped. At the end of six years he was continuing work satisfactorily and has had no relapse of symptoms in between.

Recurrent Depressive Disorder

Depression is highly recurrent and 60–70% of patients relapse within a period of five years. Half of them relapse within a year. Risk of relapse is greater if not treated.

CASE 2

Mrs. X, a 48-year-old house wife and mother of 2 children was admitted in the hospital with a history of recurrent episodes of depression since her 26th year of age. The first episode coincided with the death of her mother in law of whom the patient was very fond of. A week after her death Mrs. X woke up from her sleep telling that her mother-in-law was not really dead and had just gone to her brother's house which was on the other part of the town. She rang up to that house to enquire whether the old lady had arrived there. The relatives rushed to Mrs. X's house and found the patient weeping profusely telling repeatedly that she "knew where to search for her mother in law"! Over the next three days she slept poorly and ate little as she had no appetite. She cried most of the day, was not interested to attend on her eight-month-old child or her husband. Often she moaned that she would never be able to look after them. She was hospitalized and recovered within a month and continued medicines for about 6 months and became her normal premorbid self.

She was symptom free for the next 4 years but relapsed a few months after the second delivery. She neglected her child refused to feed the baby. Was sorrowful, sleep and appetite suffered and she had occasional ruminations of ending her life. She recovered within a month in the hospital and continued the medicines for a few months, and was lost to follow up.

She had five more relapses of depression not accounting the present episode each at intervals of 3–4 years, for which she received help from another hospital. There were no known stresses which presumably precipitated each episode including the present one. She was totally free of any symptom between two episodes.

Psychotic Symptoms in Depression

Psychotic symptoms are often present along with depressed and their content may be congruent or incongruent with the prevailing mood. In the former hallucinations and delusions relate to themes of patient's health, self-esteem, financial status and social relationship. Thus, the patient may be under a delusion that he has a not yet detected serious illness like cancer or HIV. He is convinced that he is a committed sinner worthless to live in this world any more. Delusions of poverty and persecutory delusions are other mood congruent psychotic features. Mood incongruent symptoms of psychosis are those of thought insertion, withdrawal or broadcasting or others like delusions of control whose contents are not in tune to the depressive mood. Mood incongruent psychotic features are less common than the congruent ones. Depressive stupor is a psychotic state.

Box 5.2: Other Clinical Variants of Depression

Agitated depression:
Depressive disorder where psychomotor agitation is prominent marked by such acts as fidgety movements, wringing of hands, restlessly paving up and down, etc.

Retarded depression:
Depressive disorder with psychomotor retardation marked by slowness of motion, delay in responding and relative immobility.

Depressive stupor:
Stupor represents the more severe form of retarded depression. The patient is motionless and mute and unresponsive with consciousness retained. Eyes are open and follow external objects. On recovery they are able to recall all events which happened during stuporous period.

Cyclothymia:
A persistent disorder of mood characterized by swings of mood from mild depression to mild elation apparently unrelated to the person's life events. Each mood may be stable for period lasting for a few days to a few months.

Dysthymia:
Another persistent disorder of mood characterized by longstanding mild depression with short periods of "normal" mood in between. The term dysthymia means "ill tempered".

Recurrent brief depressive disorder:
Symptoms are similar to that of a recurrent depressive disorder but duration of symptoms is brief, less than two weeks, often lasting for 2–3 days only with symptom free intervals.

Masked depression:
A variant of depressive disorder where depressive mood is less obvious. Instead, physical symptoms and other features like low energy, difficulty to concentrate, work absenteeism, quarrelsomeness, easy irritability, etc. may mask the depressive mood and constitute the presenting symptoms.

Double depression:
Major depression superimposed on dysthymia. Even after recurring from a major depressive disorder symptoms of dysthymia persist which mark the base line of the patient's mood.

CASE 3

31-year-old Mrs RV with a heavy family loading of affective disorder received help for a recurrent depressive disorder of more than 6 years duration. The first episode occurred while she was 22 years old 2 years prior to marriage. The symptoms subsided by themselves after a few days and no medical help was sought. After marriage she had three more episodes at intervals of 2–3 years within a period of seven years for which she received help from the present hospital. All of them were characterized by depression, tiredness and sleep disturbances. In particular were the persecutory ideas which were consistently present during each episode. At such times the patient expressed paranoid ideas against her husband's people, particularly his parents and an unmarried sister. Mrs RV accused that they were causing her illness by giving "unhygienic food". She avoided food prepared by them and cooked her own food. Except during the period of illness the relations between the patient and others were smooth and congenial.

Box 5.3: Some Famous People Who Suffered from Depression

Many famous people have suffered from depression. People in all walks of life whether they were rich or poor, gifted or mediocre, eminent or undistinguished have been afflicted with the illness. The list is long and includes brilliant composers like Beethoven and Mozart, renowned writers and poets like Charles Dickens, Hemingway, Leo Tolstoy, Allan Poe, Lord Byron and Keats, Politicians like Oliver Cromwell, Abraham Lincoln and Winston Churchill, celebrated artists like Michelangelo and Vincent Van Gosh and world famous scientists like Sir Isaac Newton and Sir Julian Huxley. Vincent Van Gosh slashed his right ear and on another occasion shot himself with his pistol in the agony of depression. In one study of 300 world famous men 40% had suffered from depression at some time or other during their lives. High rates for depression are accounted for writers (72%), artists (42%) composers (30%) and scientists (33%).

Dysthymia

The term dysthymic disorder was introduced in 1980 (DSM-III Classification) to indicate a longstanding (2 years or more) depressive state prevails for most of the time on almost all days.

CASE 4

The patient Joy was a 30-year-old male working as a clerk in the local high school. He was a reasonably good student but discontinued studies while studying for BA. He came to the hospital because of hs persistent feelings of "sadness" of more than 10 years duration. He was sad about almost everything in life, whatever had happened to him in the past and whatever was in store, as, for example, his job, accomplishments, friends and future. He was reluctant to marry as he "had no future". He brooded over his wasted student life telling that if he had been "a little more hardworking" he could have come out of school with flying colors. He believed his parents as well teachers, were partly to blame as they did not properly direct him. He was dissatisfied with his job as "everybody at school were bossing over him and "they were selfish and solely interested in their own affairs".

The patient said that he could not remember even a single day when he was happy and cheerful. He felt destiny was cruel to him. He resented companionship of his colleagues and avoided social get togethers. While at school he was nick-named by his friends "Sour Joy".

MANIA AND HYPOMANIA

While depression represent one end of the mood spectrum. The low one, mania and hypomania occupy the other end with morbid optimism, pressure of speech, restless overactivity and unbounded energy. Hypomania is an intermediate state between normal euphoria and mania and unlike the latter is often conducive to creativity.

Mood

There is elation and the patient states that he never felt better in life. In hypomania mood is infectious and the patient is able to instill enthusiasm on others. However, he may not be able to carry them all along because of his intolerance to criticism and suggestion from others. In mania, the mood though elevated borders on sudden irritability and vicious anger whenever he is crossed or ignored. Over friendly and over intimate the patient often intrudes on others' privacy and is inconsiderate about their feelings or rights, being self indulgent, indiscrete and impatient.

Cognition

The patient's thinking is congruent to his mood. He displays unlimited confidence in his ability and knowledge and his responses are quick and witty. He talks easily, winningly and humorously and like his confidence unlimitedly. He talks and talks and talks — and talks. He admits no mistakes and justifies his every act. Any slip in planning or execution is counteracted by a score of substitute plans to which he instantly switches over disregarding completion of any of them. He is distractible, dropping one plan after another on some pretext or other. His talk is as rapid as his thinking, copius and unchecked so that often it may be difficult to follow the sequences of thought resulting in a flight of ideas. In extreme cases talk is incoherent. Delusions are common and are of the grandiose type and also persecutory as the patient believes that he is being conspired against because others are jealous of him. Themes of delusions are incongruent to the mood in mania with psychotic symptoms.

Biological Functions

Like energy the patient's appetite is also increased. He eats heartily, often gluttonously with no respect to social conventions, belching loudly and demanding more or serving himself inconsiderate of others. Sleeps little not because he is troubled with insomnia but because he thinks sleep is a sheer waste of time. Sexual behavior is uninhibited and sexual desire is increased. Sexual promiscuity often leads to illegitimate pregnancy.

Other Behavior Changes

The hypomanic patient radiates health in every step and with his liveliness catches everybody's attention immediately. His dress and demeanour reflect his liveliness, patient preferring catchy and bright colored dresses. But in mania the appearance may be untidy and neglected due to his impatience and distractibility. Despite his high energy and enthusiasm, he achieves little due to the fleety attention. The patient squanders large sums of money in buying fancied items though they are superfluous and not needed. He wins friends easily but loses them as easily because of his intolerance and bad temper.

The following excerpts from a case sheet illustrates the behavior of a manic patient.

CASE 5

"... on entering the ward she stormed into the nursing station and slapped the security "for obstructing her way". Offered to help the nurses, she herself being one, as she had a short course in first aid in her school days. Winked at the doctor and suggested that he should change his spectacle frames as that would improve his appearance. In the wards she sang at the top of her voice and laughed aloud when asked to stop making noise. Many a time she apologized for not being in her "top form" as she was brought to the hospital most unplannedly and needlessly by her envious family members. Constantly she loved to make obscene remarks and gestures and heartily laughed at them. With patients she was very friendly and said she would help them recover fast and return home "in a whiz". She said the ward needed a facelift and offered several ready plans to improve it, the foremost being air conditioning it ...".

Psychotic Symptoms in Mania

10–20% of manic patient have psychotic symptoms similar to the first rank symptoms of schizophrenia. But these are transient and seem to disappear within days. As in depression the psychotic symptoms are mood congruent or incongruent. Affectively neutral (i.e. with no special emotional significance) delusions and hallucinations are considered mood incongruent.

Bipolar Disorder

As mentioned earlier patients who suffer from repeated manic episodes alone are rare and they have associated intervening depressive episodes. At least two affective episodes of which at least one shows elevation of mood, increased energy and activity, severe enough to disrupt routine work calls for a diagnosis of bipolar disorder. Recovery is total in between two episodes.

CASE 6

A 37-year-old Hindu male teacher stopped going to school a week after returning from a religious retreat centre where he had been for 7 days. When his wife working in the same school called him to be ready he stopped her telling that he was not going to school any more as he had been told by God that morning to go for preaching instead of teaching. The teacher, by nature shy and soft spoken had shown changes in behavior, even two weeks earlier, as reported by his colleagues afterwards. Soon after reaching the retreat centre he had proclaimed he had revelations and wanted to cry as his heart was filled with joy. He was seen telling others in the centre that he was destined to be the torch bearer of God, so that others could follow him. On reaching home he moved to another room where he slept alone without allowing his wife to share the bed. He spent more time in reading the scriptures and woke up unusually early for this purpose. Being vacation time he did not have to attend school till its reopening two months later.

The patient had two episodes of depression earlier—one shortly after his marriage and the other a year later when his father died. Both needed hospitalization as he had severe suicidal ideas on both occasions.

He was brought to the hospital the next day. He showed marked pressure of speech and expansive delusions but no hallucination.

ETIOLOGY

Biological Factors

Heredity

Affective disorder runs in families. There is strong evidence favoring genetic transmission as seen from twin studies. Concordance rate for identical twins is 70% as against 20% for fraternal twins. Genetic influence is more for bipolar disorder than for unipolar disorder and is least for dysthymic disorder. Inheritance is possibly polygenic (cumulative gene effects).

Monoamine Deficiency

Monoamines are biogenic amines responsible for neuro-transmission. They include catecholamines (dopamine, nor-adrenaline and adrenaline) and indolamines (serotonin). It is postulated that depletion of monoamines results in depression.

Box 5.4: Monoamine Hypothesis

It is postulated that monoamines which are central neurotransmitter substances have a key role in the etiology of affective disorders. The brain monoamines are the catecholamines (dopamine, norepinephrine and epinephrine) and the indoleamines (serotonin). Their relative deficiency at functionally important sites in the brain is associated with depression and an excess with mania. The evidence comes from clinical and experimental studies. Treatment with reserpine and tetrabenzine depletes monoamine stores and also causes depression. Alpha Methyl Para Tyrosine (AMPT) which interferes with catecholamine synthesis by inhibiting conversion of tyrosine to dopa causes a clinical relapse of depression in patients recovering from depression. MAO inhibitor group of drugs which increase the concentration of monoamines in the brain by preventing their intraneuronal deamination (by the enzyme monoamine oxidase) counteracts depression. Dopamine agonists like bromocryptine and psychostimulants like amphetamine which release norepinephrine from neurons provoke mania. Tryptophan and other monoamine precursors are used to treat depression with good effect. In spontaneously arising depression there is evidence of a decrease in monoamine synthesis as shown by low urinary tryptamine excretion.

Endocrinal Abnormalities

Several endocrine dysfunctions are associated with depression. Examples are hypothyroidism, Cushing's syndrome, Addison's disease, etc. Depression occurring during postpartum and menopausal periods are attributed to endocrine abnormalities.

Abnormal Sleep Architecture

It is suggested that sleep abnormalities are etiological factors in affective disorders. REM latency (time between onset of sleep and onset of Rapid Eye Movement sleep) is short in depression and REM sleep is more. Many antidepressants reduce duration of REM sleep and lengthens REM latency. Total sleep deprivation or selective REM sleep deprivation temporarily relieves depression.

Cerebral Blood Flow Changes

Reduced blood flow to certain parts of the brain is attributed as causative to depression.

Drugs

Several drugs precipitate depression, as for example, reserpine. Drugs like INH and steroids precipitate mania.

DIAGNOSIS

In typical cases, depression and mania do not pose any diagnostic difficulty. But if depressive or manic symptoms are secondary to any psychiatric or physical disorder there may be diagnostic problems. Depression may be the heralding symptom of many psychiatric or physical illness. It may be associated with several medical conditions like hypothyroidism, Addison's disease, Cushing's syndrome, Parkinsonism, etc. or with several metabolic disturbances. Uremia, hepatitis, malignancies and viral infections produce depressive symptoms. Several drugs produce manic and depressive symptoms.

Tables 5.2 and 5.3 list the diagnostic criteria according to International Classification.

DIFFERENTIAL DIAGNOSIS

Depression is to be differentiated from normal sadness, anxiety disorders, schizophrenia and organic brain disorders.

Presence of other features in depression differentiates it from normal sadness. Severity of anxiety and depressive symptoms, their course of development and presence of associated symptoms in depression help to differentiate it from anxiety disorders. Course of development of symptoms, past history if any and lack of features characteristic of schizophrenia help differentiation from schizophrenia. Careful history and examination along with relevant investigations rule out organic brain syndromes.

Manic disorders are to be differentiated from schizophrenia, organic brain syndromes and drug induced psychoses.

Table 5.2: Diagnostic guidelines for depression

The following symptoms from both lists should be present for a minimum period of two weeks:

List A	List B
Any two of the following symptoms:	Any two, or three or four (depending on severity of depression) of the following:
1. Depressed mood	1. Reduced attention and concentration
2. Lack of interest, lack of joy	2. Loss of self-esteem, self diffidence
3. Getting tired easily (easy fatigability)	3. Guilt feelings, ideas of unworthiness
	4. Pessimistic view of future
	5. Thoughts or acts of self harm
	6. Disturbances of sleep
	7. Reduced appetite

Table 5.3: Diagnostic guidelines for hypomania and mania

Several of the symptoms should be present for a minimum period of one week. Symptoms are less severe in hypomania not causing total disruption of work unlike mania:

Hypomania	Mania
mild elevation of mood, increased energy and activity, marked feelings of well being, increased sociability, talkativeness	increased sexual desire, reduced need for sleep, increased energy, pressure of speech, grandiosity excessive optimism, reduced need for sleep, elevated mood to the level of excitement, perceptual disturbances, aggressive behavior and psychotic symptoms may be present

MANAGEMENT

In many cases treatment can be provided at home but hospitalization may be needed in the following conditions:

1. When depression is severe.
2. When agitation or retardation is marked.
3. Severe biological disturbances.
4. Suicidal risk.
5. Severe excitement or other management problems in case of mania.

Box 5.5: Some Risk Factors in Suicide

History:

History of previous attempts

Family history of suicide, depression, alcohol dependence

Advanced age, unemployment, poor social ties

Associated medical conditions:

Chronic painful medical conditions

Psychiatric illness, particularly depression

Drug dependence, sleeplessness

Mental status:

Severe guilt feelings and loss of self-esteem

Suicidal ruminations

Severe helplessness and hopelessness

Planning and preparation:

Suicidal notes

Procurement and possession of lethal substances planning for the final exit—preparation of will, settlement of pending affairs, etc.

SUICIDE PLAN is a useful acronym for important risk factors for suicide:

S   Suicidal rumination

U   Unemployment

I   Intoxication

C   Chronic illnesses

I   Isolation from society

D   Depression

E   Earlier attempts

P   Planning and execution

L   Loss of self-esteem

A   Advanced age

N   Notes (on ending life)

Aims of treatment are:

1. Amelioration of symptoms

2. Treating complications if any

3. Successful rehabilitation

4. Prevention of relapses as much as possible.

DEPRESSION

Drugs

There are a large number of medicines both old and new for treating depression which are dealt in Chapter 12. Their relative merits and demerits are also discussed in that chapter. It is preferable to use a single preparation but combination of drugs may be necessary to avoid adverse effects of single drugs at a higher dosage. Antianxiety drugs and hypnotics may be necessary to control agitation and to help sleep. Antipsychotic medicines will be required if there are associated psychotic symptoms. Lithium and other mood stabilizers have a major role in therapy. Lithium augments antidepressant therapy. Thyroid supplements and stimulants (e.g. amphetamine) find place in refractory depression.

Electroconvulsive Therapy (ECT)

ECT is a valuable aid to treatment and may be lifesaving when patient is stuporous, suicidal or severely agitated.

Psychotherapeutic Measures

Psychotherapy along with antidepressants is more effective than either treatment alone. It provides emotional support, correct negative cognitions and relieve guilt feelings.

MANIA

Drugs

Neuroleptics are helpful in mania and hypomania to control excitement. Adverse effects like extrapyramidal symptoms can be prevented by addition of antiparkinsonian drugs. Lithium has a significant role in acute mania and in bipolar disorders. Other mood stabilizers are also useful. These are dealt in Chapter 12.

ECT

ECT has limited place in acute mania.

Psychotherapeutic Measures

Though they do not have a role in acute conditions they will be useful when the active symptoms are controlled and when the patient is manageable.

COURSE AND PROGNOSIS

Both depression and mania tend to recur. More than 80% patients with mania or depression have recurrences. 10–15% follow a chronic course.

Unipolar disorders start later than bipolar disorders. About a quarter of them relapse within a year. A cycle lasts for about 6 months or more. The interval between two cycles becomes shorter over the course of time and 10–20% of patients have a chronic unremitting course.

Bipolar disorder starts earlier than unipolar disorders. An episode lasts from 3–6 months with fresh episodes recurring once in 2–3 years. Over the course of time the symptom-free intervals become shorter. Bipolar II disorders have a better outcome but rapid cyclers have a poorer prognosis. Less than a fourth of bipolar disorders have a 5-year clinically symptom-free intervals.

6

Neurotic Disorders

PSYCHOSES AND NEUROSES

The terms "psychoses" and "neuroses" were used for categorizing mental illnesses till recently, till the latest revision of the two main classificatory systems (International Classification of Diseases, 10th revision in 1992 and the Diagnostic and Statistical Manual of Mental Disorders-IV revision in 1994). Till then all mental illnesses were mainly subdivided into these two major groups (neurotic and psychotic dichotomy) where psychoses encompassed all "major" mental illnesses characterized by severe symptoms like delusions and hallucinations and lack of insight. Neuroses included all "minor" mental illnesses whose symptoms were closer to normal experience like anxiety, depression or fear. When illnesses were regrouped depending on their main themes and descriptive similarity these two terms were discarded in the latest revisions of the two classificatory systems (ICD-10 and DSM-IV). Their adjectival forms, i.e. psychotic and neurotic are however still retained for descriptive purposes to denote the presence or absence of some signs and symptoms. Delusions, hallucinations, gross excitement and hyperactivity, severe psychomotor retardation, etc. are considered as psychotic symptoms. When they are present the illness is described as psychotic. Their absence is characteristic of neurotic disorders.

CLASSIFICATION

According to the International Classification (ICD–10) neurotic disorders are part of a block called "neurotic, stress related and somatoform disorders". The neurotic disorders are classified as follows:

1. Phobic anxiety disorders
   a. Agoraphobia
   b. Social phobias
   c. Specific (isolated) phobias
2. Other anxiety disorders
   a. Panic disorder
   b. Generalized anxiety disorder
   c. Mixed anxiety and depressive disorder
3. Obsessive compulsive disorder
4. Dissociative (conversion) disorders
   a. Dissociative amnesia
   b. Dissociative fugue
   c. Dissociative stupor
   d. Trance and possession disorders
   e. Dissociative motor disorders
   f. Dissociative convulsions
   g. Dissociative anesthesia and sensory loss
5. Other neurotic disorders
   a. Neurasthemia
   b. Depersonalization—derealization syndrome

The block, as its name indicates include other disorders (stress related and somatoform disorders) also. In this chapter, phobic anxiety disorders and other anxiety disorders are described under the heading anxiety disorders.

ANXIETY DISORDERS

Anxiety is a subjective feeling of apprehension, dread and trepidation, an excessive concern about the present and future accompanied by a variety of somatic and psychological manifestations. These symptoms are the resultant of arousal of the autonomic (sympathetic) system and vary in intensity and duration. Anxiety is a common symptom of many physical or psychiatric illnesses. It may occur as a primary disorder in the absence of any external stimulus and not related to any environmental situation. It differs from fear by the absence of a specific cause.

Some of the clinical manifestations of anxiety are listed in Table 6.1.

Anxiety, whether it occurs in generalized anxiety disorder, phobic or panic disorders or in association with any physical or psychiatric disorder is indistinguishable physiologically, behaviorally and subjectively. Anxiety may be continuous as in general anxiety disorder or intermittent as in phobic and panic disorders. It may be situation specific as in phobic disorders. It may be transient but severe as in panic disorders.

GENERALIZED ANXIETY DISORDERS

Generalized anxiety disorders (GADs) are the commonest psychiatric disorders and are characterized by chronic anxiety not restricted to or modified by any particular situation. It is differentiated from "normal" anxiety by its intensity, pervasiveness, difficulty in controlling and the marked distress and impairment which it causes. Patients with GADs are constantly "keyed up", keep worrying about even the most trivial matters and anticipate the worst in all their dealings. Muscle tension, irritability, insomnia and tiredness are other symptoms along with those listed in Table 6.1.

Table 6.1: Symptoms of anxiety	
PHYSICAL	
Cardiovascular	Palpitation, chest discomfort, "missed beats" rapid pulse, dizziness
Respiratory	Hyperventilation, shortness of breath choking sensation, sighing
Gastrointestinal	Dry mouth, nausea, difficulty in swallowing, "lump in the throat" sensation, epigastric sensations ("butterflies in the stomach"), dyspepsia, diarrhoea "flatulence"
Genitourinary	Urinary frequency and urgency, loss of erection, menstrual disturbances
Neuromuscular	Tremors, twitching of muscles, muscular tension, headaches, backache, tinnitus
PSYCHOLOGICAL	Apprehension, difficulty in concentrating intolerance to noise, restlessness, irritability, worry
OTHERS	Insomnia, nightmares, loss of sexual interest

Epidemiology

Prevalence in general population is 3–8%. Females are more prone. It has a high concordance rate of 80–90% in monozygotic (MZ) twins and 10–15% in dizygotic (DZ) twins.

Etiology

Biological

Genetic predisposition is evident from family and twin studies. Neurobiological mechanisms involving various neurotransmitter substances (altered levels of GABA, norepinephrine, serotonin, dopamine, etc.) and various brain systems (limbic system, locus coeruleus, prefrontal cortex, etc.) are also implicated.

Psychological

Morbid anxiety occurs in people who have a personality disorder. According to psychoanalytic theory anxiety results from intrapsychic conflicts between ego, id and superego or the outside world. Learning theories postulate that anxiety which is an unconditioned response becomes a conditioned response by association with neutral stimuli.

Sociological

Repeated and prolonged stresses in childhood and in adult life pave the way to generalized anxiety.

Diagnosis

According to ICD-10 the criteria are morbid apprehension (worry, "on edge" feeling), motor tension (inability to relax, tension headache) and autonomic over activity (tachycardia, tachypnea, etc.). These occurring on most of the days for several weeks or months in the absence of other primary illnesses (depression, phobia, etc.) suggest a diagnosis of GAD.

General anxiety disorder should be distinguished from the following conditions:
- Depressive disorder
- Schizophrenia
- Substance abuse
- Dementia

Physical illnesses like thyrotoxicosis, pheochromocytoma, hypoglycemia, epilepsy.

Treatment

Pharmacological

Several antianxiety agents are available in the market like benzodiazepines, azaspirones, β- blockers, antidepressants, etc. which are dealt in Chapter 12.

Psychological

These include the various forms of psychotherapy, behavior therapy (e.g. relaxation therapy) and cognitive therapy dealt in Chapter 12.

Course and Prognosis

Many anxiety disorders disappear within several months. Some may pursue a chronic course. Many anxiety disorders over the course of time merge with depressive disorders.

PHOBIC DISORDERS

Phobias are persistent and morbid fears of specific objects or situations outside the individual. They are morbid because:
1. The fears are irrational. The feared objects and situations do not evoke fear in normal people.
2. The fear is out of proportion and insurmountable to the patient. The patient avoids them permanently.
3. Even contemplation of the feared objects produce symptoms in the susceptible.
4. Logical explanation about innocuous nature of the objects do not relieve anxiety in the affected individual.

Classification

Phobias are conveniently grouped into three:
1. Agoraphobia
2. Social phobias
3. Isolated (specific) phobias

Agoraphobia

This refers to morbid fear of open spaces or of being away from a place of shelter (usually home). Such situations include being in public places or crowds, or places of confinement from where he cannot leave without attracting attention of others (as for example, in a cinema theater, while travelling in buses, trains etc.). Even thoughts of being in such situations precipitate severe anxiety. The patient avoids such situations and if placed there tries hard to escape to "safe" places. Over the course of time the patient becomes more and more homebound ("housebound or housewife syndrome"). Some may find relief in the company of a trusted friend while in similar situations.

Social Phobia

These refer to morbid fears of situations where the patient is likely to be observed and criticized by others. Unlike in agoraphobia, social phobias occur in small groups where there is constant interaction between the group members. The likely situations are canteens and social get togethers and involve such activities like public speaking, eating in public and interactions with members of opposite sex. This also may lead to social isolation.

Specific (Isolated) Phobias

Here, the situations are highly specific as exposure to animals, darkness, thunderstorms, etc. which the patient selectively avoids. Such fears are common in children where they are normal and which disappear spontaneously. Sometimes they are carried on to adulthood.

Clinical Features

Symptoms are the same as in generalized anxiety disorder but are intermittent and occur only in the specific situations, real or imagined. When anxiety mounts up it may resemble a panic attack. Patients successfully remain asymptomatic by avoiding the situations.

Box 6.1: Types of Phobias

Specific phobias are limited to discrete objects or situations. The objects and situations are endless and include fear of heights, closed spaces, darkness, lightening, spiders, insects, animals, snakes, riding, eating in public and what not.

According to DSM-IV classification five types of specific phobias are recognized. They are:

a. Animal type (related to animals or insects)
b. Natural environment type (as for example, storms, water, heights)
c. Blood-injection-injury type (sight of blood, or injury, receiving injection or undergoing medical procedures)
d. Situational type (as for example, driving, closed spaces, elevators, etc.)
e. Other types (fear of falling, choking, loud noises, etc.)

CASE 1

A young male aged 28 years came for consultation for his constant dread of thunderstorms. The fear cost him dearly as he lost his job as a bus driver recently, a job which he was holding for more than 6 years.

As a child he was fearful of several things—thunder and lightning, strong winds, darkness, of being alone in the house and many others—all of which left as he grew up except the fear of thunderstorms. He used to bunk classes while at school (and in the college) when there were thunder and lightening on some pretext or other. After graduation he sought several jobs but was not successful in getting one till his uncle who operated several buses in town offered him this job.

He was intensely scared of lightning without knowing why. He was not fearful of getting struck by the lightning, as he was aware that it was unlikely. He sometimes was afraid whether the dazzling streak of light might make him blind ("as occur during eclipses") but otherwise he believed that his fear was irrational and silly. He also knew that he is no more at risk then the bus passengers or who walk in the streets during a thunderstorm.

At home or away from home he became disquietened long before the actual arrival of a storm. When clouds started appearing in the sky and when the sun became faded or hidden by the clouds he became increasingly anxious. A distant peal of thunder made him panicky. While at home he would retreat to the inner- most room after closing all doors and windows and draw curtains across them so that he cannot see the flashes of lightning. He would remain there till the storm was over, terror stricken with his heart pounding. Even the thought or forecast of a thunderstorm worried him intensely.

His colleagues and the work manager initially ignored his frequent absences from work during thunderstorms in a good humoured manner. But when these became a regular affair and started affecting work schedules he was asked to leave.

Etiology

Genetic predisposition and personality are considered as etiological factors. Learning theories hold that phobias are acquired through association learning.

Course and Prognosis

Phobias that arise in childhood and are carried on to adulthood continue for several years. Those acquired in adult life have a better prognosis.

Treatment

Anxiolytic and antidepressant drugs are helpful. Beta adrenergic blockers may relieve symptoms like palpitations and tremors.

Among psychological methods of treatment behavior therapy using the exposure method of behavior therapy is useful. Relaxation training and systemic desensitization are also helpful.

PANIC DISORDER

Panic disorder is characterized by intermittent severe anxiety (panic) which is not related to any particular situation. Lack of situation specificity and the paroxysms of attack differentiate it from GAD and phobic disorder. Panic disorders are otherwise termed as episodic paroxysmal anxiety.

Clinical Features

An attack lasts for 5 to 20 minutes and rarely more. It may pass off leaving anxiety and agitation for some more time (a few hours occasionally) or may recur and subside like a wave. After an attack the patient is usually asymptomatic but may be apprehensive of a repeated attack which occurs hours or days later.

The symptoms vary but usually consist of a sudden choking sensation, breathlessness, palpitations, dizziness, paresthesiae and a sense of impending doom. Feelings of unreality (derealization or depersonalization), light headedness and vague intense apprehension are common. The symptoms come unheralded while the person is engaged in routine activities like reading a book or watching the television. He tries to flee from the scene frantically to escape from the symptoms. Suicide is a common danger during an episode.

Epidemiology

Panic attacks have a one year prevalence of 1–2% in general population with a high concordance rate among twins. Females are affected more.

Etiology

Genetic: Panic disorder is familial. Monozygotic (MZ) twins are more affected than dizygotic (DZ) twins.

Biochemical: Some chemical agents like Yohimbine and sodium lactate precipitate panic attacks in susceptible individuals. Alternatingly certain drugs selectively relieve panic symptoms. These suggest a biochemical etiology.

Hyperventilation: Voluntary overbreathing precipitates a panic attack. It is postulated that involuntary hyperventilation causes panic disorder. Inhalation of carbon dioxide also has a similar effect.

Cognitive: Cognitions of having a serious illness are more common in patients with panic disorder and are postulated as a causative factor.

Diagnosis

According to the International Classification (ICD-10) panic disorder is diagnosed if several anxiety attacks occur within a period of about a month in the absence of phobia and predictable anxiety provoking situations. Symptoms should occur in circumstances where there is no objective danger and there should not be anxiety symptoms (except for anticipatory anxiety which may be present) in between two attacks.

Panic attacks occur in generalized anxiety disorder, phobic anxiety disorder and depressive disorder. Several medical conditions give rise to symptoms simulating a panic disorder some of which are:

Hyperthyroidism	Hypothyroidism
Hyperparathyroidism	Pheochromocytoma
Mitral valve prolapse	Hypoglycemia
Paroxysmal atrial tachycardia	Temporal lobe epilepsy
Drug withdrawal	Delirium

Treatment

Antianxiety agents (diazepam, alprazolam, clonazepam) and antidepressants (SSRI, tricyclic antidepressants and MAO inhibitors) are helpful in relieving panic symptoms. These are dealt in Chapter 12. Breathing exercises control hyper-ventillation. Cognitive therapy has also been found useful.

Course and Prognosis

Panic disorder runs a chronic course and symptoms persist even after several years. However, many patients have a good social outcome.

OBSESSIVE COMPULSIVE DISORDER

The core features of the obsessive compulsive disorder (OCD) are obsessions and compulsions. In common language, these two terms are used in a rather loose manner but in clinical use they are qualified by certain criteria.

Obsession

An obsession is an unwanted mental event (as for example, a thought) that intrudes into one's consciousness causing anxiety and distress. The qualifying criteria are:
1. They come repeatedly to the person's mind against his will.
2. The individual tries to check (avoid) them without success.
3. They are usually unpleasant and produce anxiety because of their alien nature.

4. The individual recognises that they are silly and illogical but still caters them.

5. The individual becomes anxious if they are not catered.

Compulsion

Compulsions are repetitive acts or rituals which like obsessions are not entertained by the individual and are actively resisted with no success. They also fulfill the above criteria.

Epidemiology

OCD has a prevalence of 2–3% in the general population with no sex preponderance. There is high concordance for monozygotic (MZ) twins.

Clinical Features

OCD may present with obsessions, compulsive rituals or both. The onset of the disorder is around the period of adolescence or early adulthood. In more than two thirds of patients symptoms are established by the age of 25. Less than 5% develop the symptoms after the 4th decade of life

The obsessive ideas are never carried out into action but they remain as a focus of worry and guilt. Some are preoccupied with guilt and remorse that an action which he had performed in the past will have a dreaded consequence on his dear ones. To counteract its effect the patient feels compelled to perform some acts which he "knows" that they "would somehow avert the danger". An engineering student had the frightening thought that each time he attended a phone call his father would meet with an accident. To counteract happening of such an event he would count from one to ten, touch the wall and draw a cross there with his finger.

Compulsions vary from simple acts like touching one's eye to more complex ritualistic performances, as for example, folding and unfolding a dress a specific number of times before it is worn, or tying a shoelace exactly alike, say half a dozen times or locking and unlocking the door a fixed number of times. One maid servant used to feel extremely uncomfortable unless she started sweeping the floor exactly at 7 o'clock. There was a rigid pattern which she fervently followed—starting with the staircase she would move to the upstairs bed room, then the drawing room followed by the dining room and kitchen. A change in the order or missing a particular room used to upset her immensely for the rest of the day. A minor variation or a reduction in the number of times brought about anxiety which was relieved only after carrying out the ritual in its full form.

Box 6.2

Obsessions take several forms—as thought, images, ruminations, doubts or impulses. Obsessive thoughts may centre around a wide variety of topics—committing immoral acts in public, shout obscene words inside the church, pushing somebody in front of a running car or stabbing a loved family member. Most commonly the patient is caught with a mortal fear whether he would do the act but sometimes he reports of an urge to carry it out. Simultaneously, there are efforts to erase the thoughts but the thoughts recur with mounting intensity.

Obsessional ideas: Thoughts or words or phrases which repeatedly come into the patients' mind. Often these take the form of obscene or vulgar words. One of Freud's classical patients had these words coming to his mind constantly—"God-shit" and "God-swine".

Obsessional images: Visual images, not hallucinations popping up in mind against resistance. One patient had a clear image of his friend committing suicide by hanging, his body wriggling in air at the end of the rope.

Obsessional impulses: Recurrent uncontrollable urges to carry out some acts—like jumping in front of a running train.

Obsessional ruminations: Repetitive inconclusive debates on a theme going on endlessly in the patient's mind. They are not phantasies as they are unpleasant and also resisted by the patient. An example is ruminations like "Does God really exist?"

Obsessive doubts: Repeated queries about one's previous action, e.g. whether the door was locked or not; whether the mains were switched off or not.

Obsessional convictions: Thought is equated with act and assumes a magical quality. One patient while walking on the tiled floor avoided cracks in between two tiles with the conviction "step on the crack, break your mother's back".

Patients with OCD are slow in their performance. Slowness is a primary feature of the disorder which is aggravated by the long time taken to complete the rituals. The patient may not be aware of or are not concerned about this disabling symptom.

ETIOLOGY

Genetic: There is high concordance of the disorder among the monozygotic (Mz) twins than among dizygotic (DZ) twins. Some 10% of parents of patients suffering from OCD have the disorder themselves.

Brain dysfunction: Brain disorders like Sydenham's chorea and encephalitis lethargica unleash obsessional symptoms. Imaging studies of the brain show abnormal metabolic activity in some parts of the brain (orbitofrontal cortex, cingulate gyrus and caudate nucleus).

Brain serotonin levels: Low levels of brain serotonin are attributed as causative as SSRI group of drugs are helpful in treatment of OCD.

Psychological theories: Psychoanalytical and learning theories have also contributed their views on the etiology of the illness. According to the psychoanalytical theory it is fixation at the anal stage during the psychosexual development which causes the disorder. According to the learning theory it is a conditioned response where anxiety is conditioned to an environmental event. Later other neutral stimuli like words, images or thoughts became associated with the initial stimulus and anxiety is lessened.

Diagnosis

According to the International Classification (ICD-10) diagnostic guidelines are:

1. Presence of symptoms for at least two successive weeks and on most days during this period.
2. The individual recognises that the obsessional thoughts are his own.
3. Thoughts or acts (at least one thought or act) are resisted actively.
4. Thoughts, acts or images are unpleasant and repetitive.

Differential Diagnosis

OCD should be differentiated from anxiety disorders, schizophrenia and depression. The magical thinking may simulate delusions. Obsessional symptoms and depression may occur together in which case careful history taking showing the evolution and precedence of symptoms and presence of associated clinical features are helpful in differential diagnosis.

Treatment

Drugs: Some tricyclic antidepressants like Clomipramine have potent serotonin uptake blocking effects and are useful in OCD. SSRI (specific serotonin reuptake inhibitors) are also helpful due to the same reason. Anxiolytics are indicated to relieve anxiety. Antipsychotic medicines are often necessary when anxiety is severe.

Behavior therapy: Exposure, flooding, thought stop and other methods are used to treat OCD with variable success. These are dealt elsewhere. Cognitive therapy is also helpful.

Psychotherapy: Supportive psychotherapy and counselling are favored as effective methods as against dynamic and exploratory methods.

Psychosurgery: Cingulotomy is done in very resistent and severe instances when other methods of treatment fail.

Dr. Samuel Johnson, the illustrious 18th century English critic, poet, biographer, essayist and lexicographer (author of the famous Johnson's dictionary) is often quoted as a person who suffered from OCD. On entering the threshold of a house which he visited, he would pause walk up and down a specific number of steps from the door, and make whirling and twisting motions. He would then make a quick jump taking a leap over the threshold making bizarre movements with his hands. While walking on the streets, he would carefully avoid the cracks between the paving stones, not stepping on them. With his walking stick he would tap on all the lamp posts on the way. If ever he missed one, he would come back, tap it and then only proceed.

Another famous name belonging to the same category is that of Howard Hughes, the US manufacturer, aviator and motion picture producer who avoided publicity. As a child he was deadly scared of "getting infected with germs". He always sealed the doors and windows of his room with special insulations. He gave directions that all articles including food delivered to him should be properly "insulated" by wrapping them with special tissue paper. He lead a lonely life in his old age and moved from one place to another in his attempts to remain anonymous. There he lived in hotels remaining inside black curtained rooms taking a meagre diet and an excess of drugs.

COURSE AND PROGNOSIS

Many patients (60–70%) improve within a year. In others the symptoms run a fluctuating or steady chronic course— sometimes lasting for 20–30 years. Presence of precipitating factors, fluctuating course of symptoms and good social rehabilitation and lack of drop outs are indicators of a good prognosis. Childhood onset and presence of associated personality disorders indicate bad prognosis.

DISSOCIATION (CONVERSION) DISORDERS

Dissociation (conversion) disorders were earlier known as hysteria or hysterical neurosis. These two terms which have become obsolete are no more in use.

Psychiatry owes much to Freud for his studies on hysteria and on the origin and development of neurotic symptoms in general. Working with Joseph Breuer an older physician, Freud discovered that many symptoms which their patients presented with had no organic basis whatsoever. He allowed such patients to talk freely using hypnosis (to reduce internal resistance), or through "free association", a technique which he later developed. This consisted of talking "freely" whatever came to the patient's mind with no regard to logic or decency. Freud discovered that the origin of the symptom pointed to some of the patient's painful experiences in the past. The symptoms were monuments of some shocking or terrifying past events in the life of the patient of which he had no recollection whatsoever in his ordinary life. This led to the assumption of a new continent of the human mind, the subconscious (meaning below the terrain of the conscious) or unconscious (indicating that the terrain and its content are *really* unconscious or totally inaccessible to ordinary introspection). Freud formulated a topographical model of human mind with three levels of consciousness—the conscious, the preconscious and the unconscious. The conscious is the small realm of the mind that holds what people are aware of in the waking state. It represented the "tip of the iceberg", the small part above the surface of water, which alone is visible externally. The preconscious is again a small portion of mind below the conscious, storing things which are not in the conscious but which can be made easily accessible. The unconscious form the largest portion of the mind, the submerged, invisible part of the floating iceberg, which is not directly accessible to awareness. The unconscious is a realm of buried memories, a dump box of painful feelings, ideas, impulses and urges which are tied to anxiety and which the individual does not like to remember. Materials which are prohibited expression in the ordinarily life are pushed back into unconscious by a censoring mechanism, never to emerge again and disrupt normal life — this process known as repression.

Repressed materials do not lie dormant in the unconscious. They are dynamic and are constantly active. They try to get out and come to the conscious for which access is denied. However they sometimes succeed either directly or not, most often symbolically—by such manifestations as dreams, slips of the tongue, parapraxes and psychiatric symptoms like pain, paresthesiae, fits or motor weakness. These psychic events take place below the surface—in the unconscious and for a clinician are the "royal roads to unconsciousness".

The unconscious mind is a product of repression. In the infant where there is no conscious/unconscious dualism the unconscious does not exist. But as soon as he realizes that some of his actions are not approved by his parents and are forbidden the process of repression starts. These repressed materials soon start exerting influence on the actions of the infant and in his later life. The conscious and unconscious portions of the mind (the term unconscious should not to be confused with unconsciousness) differ not only in the nature of their contents but also in their working. Freud later modified his hypothesis and renamed the conscious and unconscious mechanisms by other terms like id, ego and superego.

Box 6.4: Sigmund Freud

Sigmund Freud was born on 6th May 1856 in Freiberg, a small town in Moravia, now part of (Czechoslovakia). When he was 4 years old his father, a Jewish Wool merchant moved to Vienna with his family. Freud grew up, educated and practiced there almost his entire life. In 1938, he fled to England from Nazis where he died a year later.

Freud went to Paris in 1885 to study under Charcot. He returned to Vienna and became Professor of Neurology in the Vienna University from 1902 to 1938. While in Vienna he worked on neurotic patients with an older physician, Joseph Brewer which paved the way for foundation of the psychoanalytic school.

Freud's greatest contribution to science is considered to be his concepts of an unconscious mind, and of psychic determinism. He conceived unconscious as a prison house of long forgotton repressed memories and impulses which were buried there due to their primitive and objectionable nature. These however continue to influence one's behavior in health and disease. Psychic determinism holds that behavior which is otherwise non explainable can be attributed to specific psychic determinants, as for example, the dynamic forces of the unconscious.

Freud also described a set of mental mechanisms (defence mechanisms or ego defence mechanisms) which make the neurotic behavior more comprehensible. When there are mental conflicts which are not solved at a rational level these mechanisms operate at an unconscious level making the experience less painful and often resolving the conflicts successfully. Freud said that the use of such mechanisms is universal. Today psychoanalysis is a scientific discipline with its basic propositions and theoretical functions in addition to its being a method of investigation and therapeutic techniques. Psychoanalysis apart from being a school of psychology is both a research and treatment paradigm. There are several variations of theoretical techniques. The original method as formulated by Freud is referred to as classical (Freudian) psychoanalysis.

Through repression even the most agonizing events are buried deep into the unconscious and are "forgotten". But repression is not always successful. Repression breaks down when another traumatizing event of a similar type occurs in later life leading to a "return of the repressed". A neurotic symptom is then produced. This can also occur when the censoring mechanism is partly out of commission as in the case of dreams during sleep. To use Freud's metaphor "when the watchman drowses the prisoners slip out in disguise".

During symptom formation there is however one difference. The affect (anxiety) accompanying the trauma is converted to a physical symptom, either motor (e.g. paralysis) or sensory (e.g. paresthesia). Because of this channelisation, called *dissociation* of the accompanying affect the patient is free from anxiety *(la belle indifference)*. This anxiety dissipation is called the *primary gain.* Quite often the patients are reluctant to relinquish their symptoms because with the removal of symptoms the anxiety associated with the trauma reappears. Moreover, the symptoms themselves bring forth some advantages to the patient in the form of sympathy from his friends and relatives and freedom from responsibility. This is called *secondary gain.*

One cardinal point in Freud's theory is that the origin of every neurotic symptom goes back to childhood. Successful treatment of neurosis thus involves seeking out that symptom by disinterring from the unconscious the unresolved conflict of childhood which caused the symptom. It would also involve progressive stripping off its disguises until the true identity of the "fugitive" (who escaped from the prison of unconscious) is revealed.

Clinical Features

Dissociative Amnesia

The characteristic feature of dissociative amnesia is loss of memory for important personal information which cannot be explained as due to ordinary forgetfulness. Young adults are affected more and the severity and completeness of amnesia varies from time to time and from one investigator to another. Total amnesia is rare. Amnesia also may be variable from time to time. The patient may react to his symptom with perplexity and distress but many times with a *la belle indifference*. The symptoms may pass off within days.

Dissociative Fugue

In dissociative fugues there is loss of memory as in dissociative amnesia but in addition the affected person wanders away from his home or working place. Sometimes he assumes a new identity in the new place. He lives and works normally but on "recovery" is unable to explain how he came there and has total amnesia of the intervening period.

Box 6.5: Ganser Syndrome

This is an uncommon psychiatric syndrome first described by Ganser in 1898. It is also known as the "syndrome of approximate answers" as the main clinical feature is giving approximate and wrong answers to simple and familiar questions. As for example, a patient answered that the sum of 2 + 2 is 5, that he has three eyes and 11 fingers and that there are 8 days in a week. Another patient when asked about the first day of the week said "Wednesday". A red flower was pointed out to name its color when she said it was green. She said the cow had five legs.

Four clinical features are considered as essential to the syndrome: (1) clouding of consciousness, (2) approximate answers, (3) dissociation (conversion) symptoms and (4) hallucinations. Patient may appear confused and perplexed. Answers are absurd and may be inconsistent when repeated. When pressed further the patient resorts to "Do not know" or "Cannot think properly" type of answers. Motor and sensory conversion symptom is reported. Headache, backache and other bodily symptoms are common. If hallucinations are present they are usually auditory and visual. The symptoms have a natural recovery and are self limiting unless there is an associated illness, like depression.

Differentiation of dissociative amnesia is from organic amnesias and feigning. Organic amnestic syndromes are not restricted to traumatic or personal events and are not affected by abreaction. Sensorial disturbances and clouding of consciousness and other neurological signs are usually present in organic amnesias. Blackouts due to intoxication, postepileptic amnesia and post-traumatic amnesias can be ruled out by history.

One of the most famous cases of dissociative fugue relates to that of Rev. Ansel Brown of USA. In January 1887, he boarded a tramcar after drawing a large sum of money from the bank. Meanwhile in another part of the country, some 300 km away one A J Brown rented a small grocery stall and successfully carried out his trade. One day in March 1887, Brown woke up in fright asking people in that house where he was and how he reached there. He said that his name was Ansel Brown and belonged to another part of the country. The last thing he remembered was of drawing some money from his bank.

Dissociative fugues are to be differentiated from postictal fugues seen in temporal lobe epilepsy by history and investigations.

Dissociative Stupor

In dissociation stupor the patient is mute and motionless but is aware of the surroundings as can be judged by coordinated eye movements. Muscle tone, posture and breathing are not altered. History and examination reveal no evidence of an organic cause. History of psychogenicity may be present. Dissociative stupor is to be differentiated from stupor of schizophrenia and depression through history and presence or absence of associated features.

Trance and Possession Disorders

Trance refers to a state of altered consciousness as seen in hypnosis or during periods of religious ecstasy. In possession disorder there is assumption of a distinct alternate personality as if "possessed" by a diety or spirit of a dead ancestor with or without alteration in consciousness. Both have symptoms which are culture bound. In some trance states the individual falls down to the ground, shrieks and exhibits a stereotyped set of movements or postures making utterances characteristic to the particular culture. Awareness of the surroundings is partial. On recovery the person is exhausted and may appear confused. He may report of partial amnesia of the event.

In possession syndromes the individual behaves like the assumed personality referring to himself in the third person and engaging in complex activities and vocalization which are alien to his normal self. This also may be short lived as the trance states and soon passes off with amnesia for the whole event.

Trance like states may occur secondary to schizophrenia or depression.

MOTOR AND SENSORY DISTURBANCES

Dissociative motor disturbances take the form of weakness, paralysis or abnormal movements. There may be inability to move one or all limbs and the patient may complain of inability to walk or even stand unaided. Tremors, ataxia, apraxia, dysarthria or aphonia may occur as dissociative motor symptoms.

Dissociative convulsions are another type of motor disturbances. These may simulate epileptic seizures but differ from them in several aspects. Some common differentiating features of epileptic and dissociative seizures are listed in the Table 6.2.

Table 6.2: Epileptic (true) seizures and pseudoseizures

Epileptic seizures	Dissociative seizures
i. Convulsions have a fixed pattern with tonic clonic movements and a predictable course. Short lasting	No true convulsions. The pattern changes from time to time. But an "experienced" person can simulate "true" convulsions
ii. Lasts for 30–60 seconds	Considerably prolonged — may last up to 30 minutes or more
iii. Occurs any time of the day and even during sleep	Never during sleep
iv. Tongue biting, physical injuries common	Absent. Patient is able to guard against any physical injuries
v. Urinary and fecal incontinence may accompany seizures	No incontinence
vi. Neurological signs like plantar (upgoing) and eye reflexes (pupillary and corneal) present	Not present
vii. Has amnesia of the whole event	No memory disturbances
viii. Post-ictal symptoms usual (like confusion, headache).	Absent

History (presence of stressful situation, secondary gain) and examination usually provide clues to their dissociative nature. Symptoms vary markedly over periods of time and from examiner to examiner and with suggestion. Indirect observation (without patient's knowledge that he is being observed) may often reveal that the symptoms are absent when the patient is alone or when his attention is diverted. Symptoms get aggravated in the presence of others.

Sensory disturbances take form of anaesthesiae, pain and paresthesiae not respecting the laws of innervation (socks and glove type; or over a sharply circumscribed area). Dissociative blindness, deafness or anosmia are other examples of sensory disturbances.

Diagnosis

"Hysteria" (dissociation disorder) is a great mimic and can imitate almost any illness known to mankind. In differentiation "hysterical" symptoms both positive and negative points should be taken into account.

Some diagnostic guidelines are:

1. Absence of a physical disorder which could explain the manifest symptoms.
2. Nonconfirmation to anatomical and physiological principles
3. Presence of psychogenic factors in the form of stressful events and disturbed relationship.
4. Multiplicity of discrete symptoms which cannot be accounted by a single organic pathology.
5. Presence of suspect symptoms (e.g. aphonia in a person who can cough aloud).
6. Certain behavior patterns like attention seeking behavior, tendency to exaggerate and dramatise one's symptoms and *la belle* indifference.

Practical problems arise when an organic condition coexists with dissociative disorders. Repeated examination under various conditions should be carried out in suspected instances.

Management

Acute disorders are to be managed with reassurance and suggestion. Patient should be helped to resolve stressful situations that evoked the symptom. Symptoms of longer duration need prolonged help in the form of environmental manipulations and gradual elimination of secondary gain. The therapist should encourage patient in helping himself (self help). Relatives should be reassured and prevented from providing sympathy and undue concessions as this breeds secondary gain. Antianxiety and antidepressant medicines may be needed for short periods.

OTHER NEUROTIC DISORDERS

Neurasthenia: Otherwise known as chronic fatigue syndrome neurasthenia is characterized by increased fatigue on mental effort along with persistent physical weakness and exhaustion and minimal physical effort. Dizziness, aches and pains, tension, sleep disturbances and irritability may be accompanying features. Easy fatigability and weakness are the core symptoms. **Depersonalization derealization syndrome** is another neurotic disorder. In the former the person feels that his body, activity and feelings are not his own and that he is estranged to himself. In the latter he perceives his environment as strong and unfamiliar. It has changed its quality and is unreal and artificial.

STRESS REACTIONS AND SOMATOFORM DISORDERS

According to the ICD-10 classification the block containing neurotic disorders include two more categories. They are:

1. Reactions to severe stress and adjustment disorders and
2. Somatoform disorders.

Stress reactions: An overwhelming stressful event may give rise to an acute stress reaction characterized by symptoms like "daze", depression, anxiety, anger, excitement or withdrawal. Symptoms may be mixed and changing. They resolve rapidly within hours or at the most within a couple of days. Less severe and chronic stress leads to adjustment disorders with onset within a month and the symptoms may last for several months.

Somatoform disorders. Somatoform disorders are characterized by repeated presentation of physical symptoms suggesting a physical disorder in the absence of demonstrable organic findings. The individual resorts to repeated investigations which are all negative. One type of somatoform disorder is hypochondriacal disorder. There is morbid preoccupation with some serious and progressive physical illness which the person believes that he has. Disease conviction and disease phobia characterize the condition unlike in dissociation disorder there is no *la belle* indifference and fear of an underlying illness is the prevailing mood. Such patients are afraid to take medicines for fear of their adverse effect but they repeatedly request for further investigation to rule out an illness.

7

Organic Mental Disorders

The term "organic" and "functional" are used very frequently in psychiatry. The term organic is used to describe a group of disorders with demonstrable abnormalities in the structure and function of brain. The patient's symptoms have a direct bearing to the brain dysfunction due to the cerebral pathology. Such demonstrable abnormalities are absent in functional disorders despite the fact that many of them have a neurological basis. Thus, schizophrenia and depression are not grouped under organic disorders even though they have an organic basis. Often the boundaries between organic and functional mental disorders are vague and ill defined.

Organic mental disorders constitute a large variety of clinical conditions with markedly different symptoms. The clinical manifestation depends mainly on three factors:

1. *Mode of onset:* Whether acute or chronic. This refers to the abruptness of onset of brain dysfunctioning.

2. *Extent of dysfunction:* Whether generalized or focal— Generalized dysfunction occurs when the brain is affected as a whole. Focal dysfunction occurs when the insult is localized, as for example, a localized tumor.

3. *Impairment of mental functions:* Whether global or limited to specific functions. Global impairment affects all mental functions where as specific impairment affects one or two functions selectively, as for example, mood, perception, thinking, etc. alone.

In general, these factors rather than the specificity of etiological factors decide the clinical presentation. That is, when the damage is diffuse and widespread the mental disturbance is same whether the damage is due to head injury or hypoglycemia or intoxication. Similarly, the localization or abruptness of onset rather than the causative organic factors decide its resultant symptoms.

Box 7.1

Focal brain syndromes: Selective lesions of cerebral cortex and of subcortical areas result in characteristic symptoms and signs.

Frontal lobe

Lesions bring abrupt changes in personality and behavior. Social disinhibition, over-familiarity, indulgence in puerile jokes, tactlessness and a lack of concern over future are shown. There is a callous concern for the feelings of others. Mood is euphoric but depending on the site of lesion there may be apathy and indifference with lack of spontaneity. Cognitive functions are impaired. Extension to the motor area causes paresis and motor dysphasia results when Broaca's area is involved.

Parietal lobe

Sensory disturbances and a wide variety of cognitive disturbances result from lesions of parietal lobes. Receptive dysphasias, agnosias, body image disturbances, right-left disorientation, dyscalculia, finger agnosia, agraphia and acalculia are some of the disturbances seen. Constructional and dressing apraxia occur with parietal lobe lesions. Often there is anosognosia (denial of one's disabilities).

Occipital lobe

Complex visual recognition disturbances. Agnosias include alexia without agraphia (inability to *understand written or printed material) asimultagnosia (inability to perceive visual scene as a whole), prosopagnosia (difficulty to recognise familiar faces), color agnosia and visual object agnosia (difficulty to localize objects in space).

Temporal lobe

Marked behavioral disturbances similar to frontal lobe lesions result from temporal lobe lesions also. Emotional instability, aggressive behavior and language disturbances (alexia, agraphia and sensory dysphasia) are seen. Paranoid delusions are common with right medial temporal atrophy. Memory disturbances both verbal (lesions on dominant side) and nonverbal (lesions on the non-dominant side) are prominent as well as multiple neurological signs.

Subcortical areas

Various disturbances involving memory language and mood occur in lesions of subcortical structures.

Dysfunction of the brain may be primary or secondary. In primary dysfunction, the brain is directly affected as occurs in brain injury, infections like encephalitis, degenerative changes, neoplasm, etc. In secondary dysfunctions brain is affected secondarily by factors elsewhere in the body as, for example, uremia, systemic infections and the like which occur outside the brain.

Acute brain dysfunctions are called delirium. In delirium, the brain dysfunction is generalized and impairment of mental functions is global. The cause usually lies outside the brain. Chronic brain disorders are referred to as dementia. Here also the brain dysfunction is generalized and the psychological impairment global. The cause is usually within the brain, mostly of a degenerative type.

CLASSIFICATION

The organic mental disorders are classified as follows according to the International Classification (ICD-10):

1. Dementias
2. Delirium
3. Impairment of specific mental functions due to organic dysfunction and physical diseases
4. Personality and behavior disorder due to brain dysfunction.

DEMENTIAS

Dementias are a heterogenous group of psychiatric disorders characterized by progressive and generalized impairment of intellectual functions. Memory disturbances are the most prominent but there are other cognitive deficits also in a state of full alertness. About 10% of all dementias are treatable and reversible but the majority are chronic and irreversible.

Epidemiology

Dementia is a disorder of old age and the risk increases as age advances. 0.5–1% people under 65 years of age suffer from dementia. Over the age of 85 years it is 4–5 times more frequent. 50–60% of all dementias are of the Alzheimer's type. Next in frequency are the multi-infarct dementias.

Clinical Features

The illness has an insidious onset unless it is associated with trauma or infection or aggravated in the course of another medical or social event. The beginning cannot be dated precisely. Memory disturbances are usually the earliest symptoms. The slow progress gives enough time to carry on the routine activities without much of a hindrance. The defects are attributed to "age" and "carelessness". At times a behavior which is anomalous to the patient's previous personality, may be the earliest symptom— like urinating in public or acts of sexual disinhibition.

In Alzheimer's disease (DAT) which is the most common of all dementias three phases in the course of illness can be distinguished. In the first phase, which may last for 2–3 years, failing memory is the most characteristic feature. The business-man forgets appointments or the teacher falters while teaching. The house wife misplaces things and blames the servant. Rarely there is an isolated episode where the individual shows some disorientation for time and space. He is either perplexed over this or readily cooks up a story to cover the defect. Everyday tasks became muddled up to some extent. There may be some restless hyperactivity but apart from these there is no serious abnormality which can be seen in the patient's behavior.

The next stage is marked with more rapid changes. There is more evident memory disturbances and a greater decline in day to day performances. The house wife is unable to work with the domestic tools with which till then she was well versed. There is greater evidence of personality and intellectual deterioration. Some focal neurological symptoms start appearing the exact nature of which depends on the site of damage. When the parietal lobes are affected there are agnosia, apraxia, dysphasia and acalculia. Extrapyramidal symptoms may be present. Dressing becomes problematic and the patient may insert her right arm in the left sleeve. Or the arms are inserted from the cuff end (dressing apraxia). Disorientation for time and space become marked and an everyday event. Mood becomes labile marked with catastrophic reactions (flashes of anger) when the patient fails to comply with the given instructions. But the prevailing mood is one of happiness which he tries to maintain. Psychotic symptoms may be present of a delusional or hallucinatory nature.

When dysphasia and memory loss become more severe and with greater neurological deficits the patient now enters the third phase — that of profound deterioration. He is bed ridden and doubly incontinent. There are disturbances of posture and gait when he tries to get up and walk. He is slovenly in dress and demeanour. Clothes become dirty and soiled with urine and fecal matter. Talk is fragmented and incoherent deteriorating to meaningless monosyllables. He does not recognise even his close relatives or misidentifies them, as for example, addressing wife as his mother or sister or as a stranger. Some patients have focal or generalized seizures.

CASE 1

A 53-year-old male, teacher in a local school with two more years of service to his credit was seen by the general practitioners for his increasing forgetfulness. He frequently misplaced his pen and spectacles both at home and in school necessitating their replacement with new ones. He had lost four pairs of spectacles that year itself and was not able to account how he lost them. While teaching he fumbled for the correct words and had to refer to his notes which he never used to do earlier. On one occasion he went to a wrong class and had to be guided to the real class room by the school peon. He "forgot" to correct the exercise books of his students, "forgot" to pay the canteen bills and at home he found it difficult to keep proper financial records. He had been a voracious reader earlier, a habit which he stopped completely. Over the past several months he had been writing notes to remind himself of his day to day engagements but these also did not help him. At this juncture the head master advised him to take a few weeks leave for a "medical check up" when he decided to consult his family doctor. Examination did not reveal any abnormality and he was advised to take rest and "to stop worrying".

He was unable to resume work and his wife was reluctant to send him back to work in view of the memory defects which worsened over the next few months. He frequently lost his way around and was unable to go to town and return home without help. He would get down from the bus several stops ahead unless reminded by the conductor. He continued to misplace things at home and blame his wife for these happenings.

One day some two years later he suddenly could not recall his wife's name, nor the name of his daughter who arrived that morning from abroad with her husband and two children. He could not recognize the children and when the daughter told that they were her children asked her when her marriage was. The family shocked by the new developments took him immediately to a neurologist. A routine neurologic examination revealed nothing abnormal the routine laboratory tests were also negative. CT scan of the brain however showed cortical atrophy.

His condition steadily worsened and was seen a year later in psychiatry for insomnia and behavior abnormalities. He was restless and hyperactive, disoriented to all spheres and had marked memory disturbances. At times he called his wife his mother and at other times his daughter. He said his age was "20 or something" and that he had five or six children (He had one daughter only). He could not tell what his job was or the name of the school where he had worked for more than 25 years. He was occasionally incontinent and soiled the clothes. When pressed to answer questions which he tried to evade there were quick flashes of anger.

Etiology

Causes are multiple. Some of the common causes of dementia are given in Table 7.1.

Table 7.1: Some causes of dementia	
Causes	*Examples*
Genetic	Familial, Alzheimer's disease, Huntington's chorea
Trauma	Severe isolated head injuries, repeated head injuries as occur in boxers (punch drunk syndrome)
Vascular	Single or multiple infarcts, subdural hematoma
Infections and inflammations	Encephalitis, neurosyphilis, HIV, SLE, multiple sclerosis
Metabolic	Uremia, hepatic failure, anoxia, carbon monoxide poisoning, vitamin (thiamine, B_{12}) deficiency
Endocrinal	Hypothyroidism; Cushing's syndrome, hypo-pituitarism
Neoplasm	Primary and metastatic tumors
Degenerative	Alzheimer's disease, Pick's disease, Parkinson's disease, dementia with Lewy bodies
Others	Epilepsy, alcohol, normal pressure hydrocephalus

Box 7.2: Degenerative Dementias

Alzheimer's disease: Most common of all dementias. There is generalized cortical atrophy, more severe in temporal and frontal lobes. Senile plaques and neurofibrillatory tangles are seen in the brain. Memory and cognitive disturbances are the most prominent clinical features.

Pick's disease: Less common than Alzheimer's dementia. Women are affected more and show circumscribed cortical atrophy ("Picks up cortical areas") as frontal and parietal.

Changes in character and personality (euphoria, social disinhibition) more marked than memory disturbances.

Creutzfeldt-Jakob disease: Rare disease with a rapid course. There are prominent neurological symptoms and signs (pyramidal and extrapyramidal signs and myoclonus). Highly infectious. Believed to be transmissible through tissue exudates. Brain is atrophied and spongiform. Psychotic symptoms may be present.

Huntington's chorea: Relatively rare involuntary movement disorder (chorea) with dementia which is genetically transmitted (autosomal dominant gene). It has a slow and progressive downhill course. Degenerative changes are widespread. Brain is small and atrophied with frontal lobes affected most. Subcortical structures are also affected and atrophied.

Senile dementia: Dementias in the senile age group have different causes and as age advances the causes become varied and more in number. The commonest dementia is of the Alzheimer's type which clinically resembles Alzheimer's disease. Multi-infarct dementias are also common in this age group, where there are multiple infarcts of different sizes in the brain caused by vascular pathology like embolus, arteriosclerosis, vasculitis, hemorrhage, etc.

Dementia with Lewy bodies: Lewy bodies are intracytoplasmic inclusion bodies found in nerve cells, particularly in substantia niagra of patients with Parkinson's disease. Lewy bodies, are seen in cerebral cortex also. The illness has a fluctuating course with dementia and clinical features of parkinsonism.

Diagnosis

According to the International Classification (ICD-10) the criteria for the diagnosis of dementias are:

1. Evidence of decline in both memory and thinking severe enough to disrupt routine activities of daily living.
2. Impairment of memory which affects registration, retention and recall. Immediate, recent and remote memory are affected.

3. Impairment of thinking and reasoning.
4. Duration of at least 6 months.
5. Retention of clear consciousness (unless delirium is super imposed).

Differential Diagnosis

1. **Normal ageing:** In normal ageing in spite of slowness of cognitive functioning patient's responses are accurate. New learning is possible with effort and practice.
2. **Delirium:** Sensorium is clear in dementia. It is clouded in delirium. Delirium has an acute onset and has a fluctuating course. Visual and tactile hallucinations are present in delirium. The level of attention is markedly disturbed.
3. **Mood disorders (pseudodementia):** Depression sometimes resembles dementia but in depression there is no real memory disturbance. Other depressive symptoms are present and patient can relate his problems.
4. **Amnestic disorders:** There is global impairment of all cognitive functions in dementia and not of memory alone.

Box 7.3: Amnestic Syndrome

Amnestic syndromes are characterized by the prominent impairment of recent and remote memory. Patients with such disorder are unable to recall new material (anterograde amnesia) as well as previously learnt material (retrograde amnesia). Immediate recall (tested by digit span test — repeating the numbers immediately after they are presented) is preserved. Memory is also preserved for very remote events. However, they are unable to recall events after a 5 minute distraction. There is no global intellectual impairment and attention and consciousness are not disturbed. Confabulation ("cooking up stories" to fill the memory gaps) is invariably present. Since orientation is dependent on the ability to store information on time and location it is impaired and patient might appear confused and disoriented. Most of the patient lack insight of their defects. The syndrome results from lesion of medial thalamus, adjacent midline structures and hippocampus. Onset of illness may be sudden or insidious. Acute onset results from head injuries, vascular events and toxic causes (e.g. carbon dioxide poisoning). Onset is gradual in prolonged insults to brain as chronic nutritional deficiencies, and substance use. Korsakov's psychoses seen in chronic alcoholics (due to nutritional and thiamine deficiency) is an amnestic disorder. Prognosis is generally poor in amnestic syndromes.

5. **Mental retardation:** Mental retardation is an arrested state of intellectual functioning noted during the developmental period and persist since then. Dementia develops at a later age and is a decline of previously acquired skills and intelligence.
6. **Substance abuse and medication:** A careful history helps differentiation.

INVESTIGATIONS

Routine investigations:
- Total and differential blood counts, ESR, Hb
- Urinalysis, blood glucose
- Serum electrolytes
- Renal function test
- Liver function test
- ECG

Special diagnostic tests:
- Thyroid function tests
- Serum B_{12} and foliate levels
- Serological tests for syphilis
- HIV
- Plain X-ray of skull EEG
- CT scan of brain and MRI studies

Treatment

Some 10% dementias are reversible and these should be identified and treated actively. The cause of dementia should be investigated as well as its severity and progression. The majority of dementias are irreversible and there is no curative treatment. Symptomatic measures of treatment are adopted. They may improve specific functions and reduce the rate of cognitive decline, as for example, anticholinesterase agents in DAT and dementia due to Parkinson's disease, Lewy bodies, Creutzfeldt-Jacob, disease, etc. They act through the inhibition of acetylcholinesterase (AchE) increasing the net available synaptic acetylcholine level. It is believed that dementia is associated with a decline in the levels of Ach within the cerebral cortex and basal forebrain. Donepezil (5 mg/day to start with, stepped up to 10 mg/day in 1–6 weeks), galantamine (4 mg twice a day, maximum dose 12 mg twice a day) and rivastigmine (1.5 mg twice a day, maximum dose: 6 mg twice a day) are acetylcholinesterase inhibitors available in the market. Physostigmine is a centrally active cholinesterase inhibitor (30 mg/day). The antioxidants selegeline (5–10 mg/day) and tocopherol (vitamin E 1000 IU twice a day) are said to have neuroprotective effects. Selegeline is a selective monoamine oxidase (MAO) inhibitor and increases CNS catecholamine levels.

Antipsychotics, anticonvulsants, anxiolytics and antidepressants including psychostimulants may be indicated in the management of appropriate sympoptoms. These are discussed in the chapter on Treatments in Psychiatry.

Behavioral strategies include setting up a regular daily routine, positive reinforcement and prompts and other practical aids against forgetfulness. Attention should be paid to self care and hygiene, safety and exercise as the patient is unable to look after these himself. The family care giver also requires support and psycho education.

Course and Prognosis

Except in reversible dementias the illness has a downhill course. The course of the disease may be progressive, remitting or stable for a long time. Mean survival rate is 8 years with a range of 1–20 years. Vascular dementias may show a stepladder pattern.

REVERSIBLE DEMENTIAS

Some dementias are reversible if detected early and treated promptly. Some of the treatable dementias are presented in Table 7.2.

Table 7.2: Reversible dementias	
Dementias due to metabolic causes	Uraemia, renal failure, hepatic failure, chronic hypoglycemia
Dementias due to endocrine causes	Hypothyroidism, Cushing's syndrome
Dementias due to vascular causes	Multiple strokes, subdural hematoma
Dementias due to infections	Neurosyphilis
Dementias due to vitamin deficiency	Pellagra, Korsakov's syndrome
Dementias due to some neoplasms	Intracranial space occupying lesions
Others	Normal pressure hydrocephalus

DELIRIUM

Unlike dementia delirium is an acute organic condition denoting a temporary and reversible dysfunction of the brain. The most salient feature is a clouding (but not total unawareness as in coma) of consciousness which fluctuates constantly associated with perceptual and mood disturbances. Causes are multiple and heterogeneous.

Clinical Features

Any patient with evident physiological or biochemical disturbances and who is unable to recount his symptoms properly or who is poorly co-operating for the examination should be considered potentially delirious. The patient is "confused" though its intensity and duration vary markedly and change over the course of time. The intensity of delirium is measured in terms of the level of consciousness.

Attention and concentration are difficult to arouse and sustain and the patient is easily distracted by stimuli outside or by his own internal stimuli. Details of the environment are poorly grasped or erroneously perceived. He is disoriented to time, place and new people and insists that he is in his own home, but at the same time asks about his whereabouts. The patient in the next bed is misidentified as his next door neighbour, though he is able to recognize the latter when he comes to visit the patient in the hospital. Memory is impaired and the patient would repetitively ask the same question again and again, as for example, regarding his whereabouts. Memory for immediate and recent past, events are disturbed more but memory for remote events also may be affected. Perseveration may be present, the patient repeating the same motor act again and again. Miming his routine work or habit is common (as for example, rolling a "beedi" or lighting it with an imaginary match or driving the car). Mood is variable and changing, the most common being fear, anxiety, perplexity or panic. Some patients or one patient at one time or other are quiet and depressed or even jovial. Illusions and hallucinations are invariably present. Spots on the bed sheet are perceived as bugs or other insects which he tries to pick up constantly. Markings on the wall are perceived as snakes crawling or sound of the rolling trolleys as claps of thunder. Hallucinations are most often visual though they can occur in other modalities also. Delusions, usually paranoid in nature may be present. Judgment is poor and the patient has no insight about his condition.

The symptoms and signs vary from day to day, time to time and moment to moment. This fluctuation of symptoms with intervening "lucid intervals" are characteristic of delirium. All symptoms are worse at night. Sleep is disturbed and there is usually a reversal of sleep-wake rhythm.

CASE 2

The patient was a 55-year-old carpenter who had been taking country liquor excessively for the past eight years after his wife deserted him. He was admitted in the wards four days ago after a blackout during which he tried to burn his house. He was prevented from doing this by his neighbor who took him to the hospital. Patient had no memory whatsoever of his action the next day of arrival in the hospital.

On the third day of his arrival he complained of "shakes" all over, particularly hands because of which he was unable to hold any objects. He found it difficult to drink from a cup as he could not hold the cup. He complained of intense fear that he would fall down from the cot and grasped the sides of the cot tightly. He had difficulty in sleeping which was fitful and interrupted. He woke up frequently with jerks of the whole body.

When seen in the wards the patient was "confused" and perplexed. He was grossly disoriented and at times said that he was in his home and at others that he was in town where he had been working irregularly. Sometimes he asked where he was lying and how he reached there. He looked vacantly at the doctor and nurse and did not appear to recognize the surroundings. Apart from these and tremors of hands he had no gross disturbances.

When seen at night on the same day the patient was agitated and terror stricken. He was unable to stay on his bed and tried repeatedly to slip down and run away because of which he had to be physically restrained. He looked at the people around him fearfully. He was very distractible, could not comprehend or answer even very simple questions. He periodically called out the names of his family members. Waved arms in the air as if to catch something and examined it carefully after opening the fist, searching for and picking up something from the open palm. Did not speak but rambled incoherently to the questions asked. He seemed to be hallucinating by the constant gazing at space with wide open eyes which he shifted as if tracking the object there. His attention was so fleety that a moment after his name was called—to which he responded by looking at the doctor—he was lost to himself. His consciousness drifted in and out at varying levels through out the night.

ETIOLOGY

The causes, as in dementia, are multiple. Table 7.3 lists some of the common causes of delirium.

Risk Factors in Delirium

Several risk factors have been identified as predisposing to delirium. Four important risk factors are preexisting cognitive impairment, visual defects, severe medical illness and dehydration. Some others are aging, malnutrition, polypharmacy, anticholinergic medication, fatigue, substance abuse, history of head injury, sleep deprivation and individual susceptibility.

Table 7.3: Common causes of delirium	
Trauma	Head Injury
Infections	Systemic infections, exanthema, septicemia, intracranial infections as meningitis, encephalitis
Metabolic causes	Hypoxia, hypercapnea, hepatic failure and precoma, uremia, cardiac failure, water and electrolyte imbalance
Endocrine causes	Hypoglycemia, diabetic precoma, hypopituitarism hypo- and hyperthyroidism
Vascular causes	Circulatory disturbances, sub arachnoid hemorrhage, CVA (acute phase)
Substance abuse and drugs	Alcohol, barbiturates, digitalis, dopa, anticholingergics anticonvulsants, opiates, annabis, steroids
Others	Epilepsy, vitamin deficiency (B_1, B_6, B_{12}), sensory deprivation, withdrawal state, postoperative states (including ICU delirium) sleep deprivation

Diagnosis

Diagnosis is clinical though investigations (like EEG) will confirm the diagnosis and define the etiology. According to the International Classification (ICD-10) all the following are necessary for a definite diagnosis of delirium:

1. Impairment of consciousness and attention.
2. Global cognitive disturbances – disturbances in orientation, perception (illusions and hallucinations), thinking (incoherence, loss of abstraction, delusions) and memory.
3. Psychomotor disturbances (hypo- or hyperactivity with shifts from one to the other.
4. Sleep disturbances, reversal of sleep wake rhythm.
5. Mood disturbances (fear, anxiety, perplexity, depression, etc.).

Delirium should be differentiated from acute psychotic disorders and acute schizophrenia or acute mood disorder with confusional symptoms. It also should be differentiated from dementia.

Investigations

A thorough history is essential which provides further clues to the areas of investigation. A medication review and a neurological examination are also equally important. Laboratory investigations include:

- Total and differential blood count
- Urinalysis
- Serum electrolytes, blood urea and creatinine
- Blood sugar
- Liver function tests
- CSF examination when necessary
- Chest X-ray, ECG, EEG and CT scan when necessary.

Electroencephalogram (EEG) facilitates diagnosis of delirium and detects minor degrees of impairment of consciousness.

Treatment

Early diagnosis and treatment are imperative as delirium is a medical emergency and often life-threatening.

Among drugs haloperidol is considered as a first line agent though other antipsychotics are also used to control the excitement and as disease specific. Minor tranquilizers control agitation and are given along with hypnotics to ensure sleep. Anticonvulsants may be necessary for patients who are at risk.

Patients are preferably hospitalized even in milder forms of delirium. In severe cases admission in intensive care units may be needed. Patient should be nursed in an environment with optimum sensory stimuli. Too much or too little stimulation may be harmful. Soft physical restraints may be needed when intensely agitated or restless. It is ideal to have the same set of staff to attend on the patient. Measures to reorient and to enhance communication and to reinforce cognitive functions are helpful which can be carried out by the attending persons with whom patient is familiar.

Preventive Measures Against Delirium

Some measures, both pharmacological and nonpharmacological are advocated for those who are at risk to develop delirium. These include specific protocols against specific risk factors as for example, orientation protocol for cognitive impairment (reorientation tasks as repeated discussion of current events, etc.) sleep protocol (milk at bedtime, relaxation, quiet surroundings, etc.), dehydration protocol (oral rehydration), sensory protocols (visual aids, amplifying devices, etc.) and early mobilization protocol. Pharmacological preventions include low dose antipsychotics, supplemental oxygen, correction of hypoxia, electrolyte imbalances and anemia.

Course and Prognosis

Delirium usually lasts for 3–7 days though it can persist for 3–4 weeks. When properly treated most of the deliria resolve completely but some may resolve only gradually and incompletely and move into a permanent cognitive disorder. Without adequate treatment it has a high mortality (5–6% death rate for delirious patients according to one study). "Hyperactive" delirious patients have a better outcome than "hypoactive" ones.

8

Disorders of Personality

There are few terms in psychiatry which are more mis-understood than personality. In colloquial language the term is used (wrongly) to denote physical charm, attractiveness or ability to impress others. Those who lack these are dubbed as having no personality. As we shall see presently personality is a term used to denote the unique pattern of a person's make up with his individual characteristics. It is impossible to conceive him without these characteristics. To say that one has "no personality" is as illogical as saying that he has no height or weight.

Personality has been described as an enduring pattern of behavior shown in the way how an individual perceives, thinks about and relates to his environment and self. It includes his characteristic ways of conducting himself not only in every day situations but also in stresses, as well as his constitutional factors like physique, appearance, intelligence, aptitudes and character. All these make up the person's total quality, the sum total of his physical, physiological, psychological and behavioral characteristics. The individual constituents or characteristics of personality are called traits. An individual is a bundle of characteristics or traits with an integrated pattern which is unique to himself. Personality may be defined as an integrated pattern of traits.

Traits are theoretically countless in number. Any adjective used to qualify a person would turn out to be a personality trait—whether this relates to the person's physique, intelligence, interests, attitudes or any other attribute. Traits do not imply abnormality. They are labeled abnormal only when they affect social functioning causing distress either to self or to the society.

Assessment of personality is a routine step during clinical examinations. It serves several purposes: (i) It identifies the uniqueness of the individual and how he stands out from others, (ii) personality modifies the clinical features of an illness, (iii) it gives an idea how the person will react to a stress or illness, (iv) it also helps prediction of the outcome of treatment as certain personality disorders worsen the prognosis when they coexist with the illness.

PERSONALITY, PERSONALITY CHANGE AND PERSONALITY DISORDERS

Personality, personality change and personality disorders should be differentiated from each other. As mentioned earlier personality is an integrated pattern of traits which are numerous and whose presence does not imply abnormality. It is also defined as "the characteristics that lead people of similar intelligence and knowledge when placed in similar circumstances, to react in different ways". They are exhibited, and therefore, assessed in a wide range of social and personal contexts, as described in the chapter on case taking. Consider the following examples.

"........*she was a dear little creature with such a smiling tender, generous heart that everybody loved her. Her eyes glowed with kindness and good humour, except indeed when they filled with tears, and that was a great deal too often. The gentle little thing would cry over a dead bird; or over a mouse that the cat had killed; or over the end of a novel, if it was sad. If anyone said an unkind word to her, she burst into tears at once*" (Vanity fair — H.M. Thackeray, retold by E.F. Dodd, Macmillan's stories to remember).

".......*he came a tall, strong heavy, nut brown man; his tarry pigtail falling over the shoulders of his soiled blue coat; his hands ragged and scarred, with black broken nails; and the sabre cut across one cheek, a dirty, livid white; a silent man by custom, all day he hung around the cove, or upon the cliffs, with a brass telescope; all evening he sat in a corner of the parlor next the fire and drank rum and water very strong. Mostly he would not speak when spoken to; only look up suddenly and fiercely and blow through his nose like a fog-horn*" (Treasure island — R.L. Stevenson).

Personality disorders like personality are stable and long-standing patterns of behavior and are developmental conditions, appearing in childhood or adolescence and carried into adulthood. They are pathological because:

1. They are inflexible and maladaptive.
2. They are an enduring pattern of attitudes and behavior which are markedly disharmonious and deviant from the expectations of the individual's culture.
3. They cause functional impairment and or subjective distress.

In contrast to the above, personality change is acquired in later life in response to stressful events or illnesses which include:

1. Injury or organic diseases of the brain.
2. Diseases of the endocrine system.
3. Systemic diseases which may also affect the brain.
4. Substance abuse.
5. Environmental deprivation.

PERSONALITY DISORDERS

According to International Classification of Diseases (ICD-10) specific personality disorders (F 60) are included in a wider block (F60-69) which contains in addition other conditions and persistent behavior patterns found in adult life. According to DSM-IV all personality disorders are listed in a separate section (code 301).

Classification

In ICD-10 eight specific personality disorders are listed which are as follows:

a. Paranoid personality disorder
b. Schizoid personality disorder
c. Dissocial personality disorder
d. Emotionally unstable personality disorder with two types:
   i. Impulsive type
   ii. Borderline type
e. Histrionic personality disorder
f. Anankastic personality disorder
g. Anxious (avoidant personality disorder)
h. Dependent personality disorder

In DSM-IV ten personality disorders are listed which are grouped in three clusters:

1. Cluster A: Baranoid, schizoid and schizotypal.
2. Cluster B: Antisocial, borderline, histrionic and narcissistic.
3. Cluster C: Avoidant, dependent and obsessive compulsive.

Comparison of classification systems of DSM-IV and ICD-10 is given in Table 8.1.

Table 8.1: Classification of personality disorders

DSM-IV	ICD-10
Cluster A	
Paranoid	Paranoid
Schizoid	Schizoid
Schizotypal	Comparable to the schizotypal behavior (F21) listed under schizophrenia Schizotypal and delusional disorders
Cluster B	
Antisocial	Dissocial
Borderline	Borderline type (emotionally unstable)
Histrionic	Histrionic
Narcissistic	No corresponding category
Cluster C	
Avoidant	Anxious
. Dependent	Dependent
Obsessive compulsive	Anankastic
No corresponding category	Impulsive type (emotionally unstable)

EPIDEMIOLOGY

Personality disorders are common. Prevalence rates vary depending on the criteria and instruments used in different studies. Many studies report overall prevalence rates (sum of all types of disorders) ranging from 10–15%. Individual rates vary, those of cluster A disorders ranging from 0.5 to 1%, cluster B from 1.5 to 2% and cluster C from 1 to 1.5%. Some types of personality disorders are more common among males (e.g. paranoid, antisocial) whereas others are more common among females (e.g. dependent, histrionic).

Clinical Features

Paranoid Personality Disorder

The most characteristic feature of people with this disorder is suspiciousness and generalized mistrust against people around him. They search for hidden meanings in their words or deeds. Neutral or friendly actions are taken as hostile and contemptuous. They bear grudges for a long time and do not forgive insults whether real or imagined. They are extremely sensitive to rebuffs and criticisms and turn litigious or combative with their strong sense of personal rights. Other features are their elevated, often unjustified feeling of self importance and tendency to blame others for their "conspiracy" in preventing them from achieving their potential. Sexual jealousy and suspicions about the fidelity of their spouses are common. Secretive and guarded, they do not mix easily in a group and do not make or retain intimate friends.

Schizoid Personality Disorder

People with schizoid personality disorder are withdrawn and reclusive and prefer solitary activities and working alone. They are emotionally cold and detached. In extreme cases, they appear callous and insensitive. They find it difficult to accept or give warm and tender feelings and are indifferent to praise or criticism. Indulge more often in phantasy life and are more introspective. Often they fail to make intimate relationships. Many prefer to live alone without marrying.

Schizotypal

Schizotypal disorder is not described as a specific personality disorder according to the International Classification (ICD-10). It is described as a separate category under schizophrenia to denote a disorder characterized by eccentric behavior and anomalies of thinking and affect resembling schizophrenia, but without any of its typical features.

The disorder is characterized by odd and eccentric behavior, preoccupation with bizarre fantasies and magical thinking that influences behavior, as for example, unusual telepathic and clairvoyant experiences. Talk is vague and circumstantial without being grossly incoherent as in schizophrenia. Paranoid ideas may be present. Affect is constricted. Perceptual disturbances include somatic hallucinations, depersonalization and derealization. They are ill at ease with strangers and even in a familiar company and keep away from them telling that they do not "fit in" the group.

Characteristic Features of Cluster A Personality Disorders		
Paranoid personality disorder	Schizoid personality disorder	Schizotypal personality disorder
Suspicion and mistrustful; bearing grudges persistently; non forgiving; resentful; excessively sensitive; sexual jealousy.	Detached and seclusive; emotionally cold; introspective; indifferent to praise and criticism preoccupation with fantasy	Eccentric behaviour preoccupation with paranormal and magical phenomenon; oddities of speech; social anxiety; unusual perceptual experiences

Dissocial Personality Disorder

Otherwise known as antisocial personality, psychopathy or sociopathy, the characteristic feature of this disorder is a callous unconcern for social norms, law or the rights of others. They are deceitful and manipulative and use any means to seek personal profits and satisfy their wishes having no guilt or remorse over the methods used. Unlawful acts are committed and often they cross swords with law and are penalized. But they do not learn from experience and continue to indulge in similar activities. Enduring relationships are not maintained. They are impulsive, act on the spur of the moment, without consideration of the consequences of their action. The frustration threshold is low as well as the threshold for violent and aggressive action. Acts of physical fights and aggression are common. Most of them have a childhood history of conduct disorders which are carried into adulthood like cruelty to animals, stealing, truancy, etc. They have a reckless regard for the safety of others or of themselves as shown by behavior such as reckless driving

Emotionally Unstable Personality Disorder

In ICD-10, this includes two subcategories—the impulsive type and the borderline type. In DSM-IV classification, there is no corresponding category to the impulsive type whereas the borderline type is represented in the same name in cluster B.

Impulsive Type

Lack of impulse control characterizes the disorder. They are moved to sudden acts of aggression and violence when provoked of which they regret afterwards. Physical violence with serious harm is common.

Borderline Type

Impulsive behavior and difficulty to control anger are described as additional features of borderline personality in DSM-IV along with other features which are shared commonly by the two classification systems. These include disturbances of identity (vague or uncertain self image), chronic feelings of "emptiness" and intense unstable relationships with others. Suicide threats to avoid abandonment and acts of self harm during emotional crises are often made.

Histrionic Personality Disorder

Self-dramatization, craving for attention from people around, exaggerated expression of emotions and self-centredness mark histrionic personality. They are excessively preoccupied with physical attractiveness and appear seductive and flirtatious. But their affect is shallow and labile as well as short lived. They seek new pastures of excitement, are easily bored and shift from one activity to another as their enthusiasm is short lived and fluctuating. People with this disorder are very suggestible and are easily carried away by the opinion of others. Though sexually provocative they turn out to be cold and frigid.

Narcissistic Personality Disorder

ICD-10 does not recognize this subcategory but DSM-IV includes it as one of the cluster B personality disorders.

People with narcissistic personality disorder are boastful and snobbish and believe that they are specially privileged and important in the society. They overestimate their accomplishments while underestimating those of others. They carry with them fantasies of their unlimited power and abilities and expect other people to acknowledge this. They seek constant attention and admiration as they believe that they deserve it. People with this personality may appear haughty and arrogant and are choosy in the relationships—as they disdain to mix with "ordinary" people.

Characteristic Features of Cluster B Personality Disorder		
Antisocial personality disorder	*Borderline personality disorder*	*Histrionic personality disorder*
Deceitful and selfish; lack of guilt and remorse; impulsive and reckless; callous, irresponsible; not learning from experience.	Disturbances of self image and identity; unstable relationships; impulsive; affective instability; feelings of "emptiness"; recurrent suicidal threats and acts of self harm to avoid abandonment	Attention seeking behavior; self-dramatization and theatricality; shallow and labile affect; self-centredness; easy suggestibility; seductive and flirtatious

Anankastic Personality Disorder

Otherwise known as obsessive compulsive personality disorder (DSM-IV) this is characterized by excessive preoccupation with orderliness, perfectionism and inflexibility. Neat and meticulous in performance, people with this disorder give pain-taking attention to minute details of a task at the cost of time and efficiency. A change of routine upsets them and they adapt poorly to sudden new situations. They dislike being "casual" and with their self imposed work discipline expect others to conform their way of doing things. There is no "time to waste" and leisure activities and friendships are postponed or excluded. They have a high sense of morality and ethics, are pedantic and conventional. Hoarding things is common, though the hoarded things are of little value. Frugal and miserly they save "for any unforeseen catastrophes in future" and disdain from luxuries of any sort even if these are affordable.

Anxious (Avoidant) Personality Disorder

People with an avoidant personality disorder are persistently tense and apprehensive. They avoid interaction with others particularly strangers for fear of rejection and disapproval and not because of emotional coldness. Feeling of inferiority and fear of social ineptness make them insecure and timid. They are unwilling to take risks for fear of failure and they restrict their life styles in order to be secure physically. They avoid group activities unless they have ample support from others. They tend to be shy, quiet and inhibited and prefer to be in the background to avoid people's attention.

Dependent Personality Disorder

This is characterized by a submissive clinging behavior and morbid dependence on others. People with this disorder have difficulty in making day-to-day decisions, as for example, the type of dress which they should wear and encourage others to make such decisions. They are afraid of being left alone or abandoned by their protectors and feel helpless in their absence. They seek an alternate source of help and protection when a close relation ends as by separation without which they are unable to care for themselves independently.

Characteristic Features of Cluster C Personality Disorders		
Anankastic personality disorder	*Anxious personality disorder*	*Dependent personality disorder*
Perfectionism	Persistent feelings of tension and apprehension	Extreme dependence on others
Marked preoccupation with details		Inability to make independent decisions
Excessive orderliness	Believes that he is socially inept and inferior	Fear of abandonment
Rigid and stubborn		
Over conscientious	Excessive fear of criticism and rejection	
Excess devotion to work so as to avoid leisure and pleasantries	Afraid to take risks for fear of failure	
Frugal and miserly	Avoids group activities unless amply supported	
Tendency to hoard things		

Etiology

No single cause is attributed as responsible to any of the personality disorders. The current view is that etiology is multifactorial with the various factors interacting and modified by social learning. Genetic, constitutional and psychological factors interplay in the genesis of personality disorders.

Genetic

Genetic factors are implicated in some personality disorders more than in others. As for example, twin and adoption studies indicate that there is heritability in antisocial and obsessive personality disorders. Many studies show that some personality disorders (paranoid, schizoid and schizotypal) are more in first degree relatives of probands with schizophrenia and delusional disorders and borderline personality disorder more in relatives of probands with affective disorders. Several traits (e.g. introversion) are heritable, this probably accounting for the personality disorders with such traits.

Constitutional Factors

Children with minimal brain dysfunction, brain injury and delay in the development of brain are at a higher risk of developing personality disorders in later life. Abnormalities of neurotransmitter transmission are correlated with some disorders, as for example, serotogenic involvement in aggressive and impulsive behavior.

Psychological Factors

Parental deprivation, criticisms, excessive parental control, humiliation and physical (particularly sexual) abuse mark early childhood years of many who in adulthood present with personality disorders. Inconsistent parenting, insecurity, cold and neglectful relations and inadequate child-mother relations have been implicated in many instances. Disorders of psychosexual development (as for example, during oral, anal and oedipal stages resulting in dependent, obsessional and histrionic personality disorders, respectively) are accounted as etiological factors according to psychoanalysts. According to learning and cognitive theories, personality disorders are due to faulty learning as by growing up in faulty environment (e.g. antisocial family), and due to faulty cognitions—incorrect evaluation of self-esteem and fear of rejection.

Diagnosis

There are no biological markers for personality disorders and diagnosis is on clinical grounds. Personality disorder is diagnosed only when the characteristic pattern: (i) develops during adolescence or adulthood, (ii) persists since then as an enduring stable pattern of the individual's long-term functioning, and (iii) does not appear only episodically or along with another mental disorder. It may be difficult to differentiate the disorder from another primary mental disorder which had an early onset and runs a stable chronic course. A personality disorder may coexist with another primary mental disorder. Personality disorder should be differentiated from personality traits. Traits do not reach the severity of a personality disorder and are not be maladaptive or cause functional impairment. Personality disorders should also be differentiated from personality change.

Course and Prognosis

Since personality disorders are defined as stable enduring patterns of behavior they persist throughout life with little change. However, over the course of time, they may become less problematic. According to some studies schizotypal disorders have the poorest prognosis whereas the cluster C disorders (avoidant, dependent and anankastic) have a better outcome.

Management

Before treatment plans are made the patient should be assessed for his strengths and weaknesses. Favorable features include compliance to treatment, motivation, conducive environment, lack of co-morbidity, etc. Strengths should be utilized and reinforced during treatment. Unfavorable features include co-morbidity, as for example, drug abuse and presence of other psychiatric disorders. While assessing environment attempts should be made to define circumstances which provoke undesirable behavior so that they can be avoided during management. Plans of treatment consist of (i) finding alternate modes of life which provoke less conflicts to the patient, (ii) avoid factors which provoke undesirable behavior, and (iii) treat and manage comorbid conditions like affective disorders, alcoholism, etc.

Antipsychotics have been used in antisocial and borderline personality disorders. Antidepressant drugs have also found limited value in several disorders. Mood stabilizers like lithium salts and carbamazepine reduce anger and impulsiveness and control aggressive and violent behavior. Habit forming drugs should be used with caution.

Psychological methods of treatment include counselling, dynamic psychotherapy and cognitive therapy. Drugs are given along with psychological methods of therapy.

Treatment is prolonged, over years. In general, people with personality disorders are poorly compliant to treatment and the drop out rates are high.

OTHER DISORDERS OF ADULT PERSONALITY AND BEHAVIOR

In the International Classification of Disorders the block containing specific personality disorders include some other related categories like personality changes, habit and impulsive disorders, psychosexual disorders and factitious disorders. Mention has already been made regarding enduring personality changes. Habit and impulsive disorders are characterized by repeated acts without any clear motivation and which harm the interests of others as well as the performer. These include such acts as pathological gambling, pathological stealing (kleptomania) pathological fire setting, etc. Sexual disorders include gender identity disorders (e.g. transsexualism, a desire to live and be accepted as a member of the opposite sex), disorders of sexual preference (Box 8.1) and those associated with sexual development and orientation (e.g. homosexuality).

Factitious disorders are characterized by symptoms which are simulated by the individual in the absence of a confirmed physical or mental disorder. The patient feigns illness repeatedly and consistently and may present in the surgery for help with self inflicted injuries. There is no secondary gain unlike in malingering, where symptoms are reported intentionally and consciously in order to accomplish a specific goal, as for example, to evade prosecutions or receive insurance claims. Factitious disorder is considered as an illness behavior but malingering is not considered as a personality disorder.

Box 8.1: Disorders of Sexual Preference

These are also called as paraphilias and include:

i. **Fetishism:** achievement of sexual excitement and gratification through "fetishes"—inanimate objects, like shoes, hair, garments, etc. A fetishist may have more than one object of adoration.

ii. **Transvestism:** Sexual gratification obtained through wearing clothes of the opposite sex.

iii. **Pedophilia:** Preferential or exclusive sexual gratification derived from children.

iv. **Bestiality (zoophilia):** Sexual gratification achieved through animals.

v. **Narcoophilia:** Erotic arousal provided by a dead body.

vi. **Exhibitionism:** Exposure of one's genital organs in front of others with a sexual intent.

vii. **Voyeurism:** Voyeurs ("peeping toms") achieve sexual arousal through watching sexual activity or body parts of other people.

viii. **Sadism:** Sexual pleasure received through inflicting pain on the partner.

ix. **Masochism:** Sexual arousal achieved through pain inflicted on him by the partner.

x. **Fortteurism:** Rubbing against or fondling the body parts of another person, usually of the opposite sex and deriving sexual pleasure.

9

Drug Dependence

A drug is any substance, natural or synthetic which has a recreational or medical value and also has the potential to be misused or abused. Thus alcohol, tobacco, morphine and LSD are all "drugs". Addiction refers to the compulsive desire to use the substance at all costs in the face of severe negative consequences. The term "drug addiction" was replaced by "drug dependence" in 1964 by the expert committee under WHO. But the term "addict" and "addiction" continue to be used in common languages even now.

Box 9.1: Use, Misuse, Harmful use and Abuse

Use: Use is a nonspecific term without implying any maladaptiveness in the consumption pattern or its deleterious effects.

Misuse: Misuse refers to overzealous or indiscrete administration of drugs (by physicians).

Harmful use: Harmful use is a pattern of use that is already causing damage to health either physical (e.g. hepatitis) or mental (e.g. depression).

Abuse: Maladaptive pattern of substance abuse, not amounting to dependence resulting in: (i) failure to fulfill social and personal obligations, and (ii) causing physical hazards (e.g. in driving the car), legal problems (e.g. arrests) or interpersonal problems (e.g. physical fights and arguments after getting intoxicated).

DEPENDENCE

Dependence is a maladaptive pattern of substance use characterized by a cluster of cognitive, behavioral and physiological symptoms. Three or more of the following criteria should be present to make a definite diagnosis of dependence.

1. *Craving:* An overpowering desire to use the substance
2. *Inability to restrict* its use and quantity
3. *Withdrawal symptoms* when the substance is not taken or if its amount is reduced
4. *Tolerance* shown by a need of taking progressively higher doses to obtain the same effect
5. *Increased preoccupation* with ways of procuring the substance
6. *Tendency to use it for longer periods* of time and in higher amounts than was intended
7. *Neglect* of social and personal obligations
8. *Continued indulgence* in spite of the real or potential health hazards of which the individual is fully aware.

CLASSIFICATION

According to International Classification (ICD-10), the substances involved are categorized in nine categories as listed in Table 9.1.

Table 9.1: Drugs of dependence According to ICD-10

Category	Examples
1. Alcohol	Beer, wine, fortified wine, spirits
2. Opioids	Opium, morphine, heroin, codeine, methadone, pethidine
3. Cannabinoids	Cannabis and its preparations (ganja, charas, etc.)
4. Sedatives and hypnotics	Benzodiazepines (diazepam), diphenylmethane (hydroxyzine) propanedioles, barbiturates, nonbarbiturates, etc.
5. Cocaine	Cocaine
6. Other stimulants including caffeine	Caffeine, amphetamines and related compound
7. Hallucinogens	LSD, mescaline, etc.
8. Tobacco	Tobacco
9. Volatile solvents	Petrol, aerosols, paints, etc.

Availability of these substances is restricted by government through licensing (e.g. opium) legislation (declaring that possession of certain cases of drugs is illegal, e.g. cocaine) routing their accessibility through prescription by a medical practitioner (e.g. pethidine) and by high taxation (e.g. tobacco, alcohol).

If three or more substances (excluding caffeine and nicotine) are used concurrently over a 12-month period, the term multiple drug abuse (poly substance abuse) is used to describe the condition.

GENERAL ETIOLOGY

Etiology is multifactorial and the different factors interact each other. Genetic, constitutional, psychological and environmental factors are attributed as causative.

Genetic

Twin and adoption studies indicate higher vulnerability to drug dependence in monozygotic (MZ) twins and adopted children of drug dependent (particularly alcohol) parents living away. Cross dependence to other substances is common. With respect to alcohol two groups have been identified—familial and non-familial alcoholics. In the former, genetic predisposition is prominent. Symptoms are massive and the onset is at a younger age group. It is also associated with an antisocial personality.

Co-morbidity: There is higher prevalence of other psychiatric disorders including personality disorders in those who are prone to drug dependence.

Brain reward mechanisms: There are biological mechanisms which perpetuate dependence on drugs once it is established. Specific areas in brain are involved in the production of craving for the substance which positively reinforce the habit by sending pleasurable signals producing euphoria and analgesia (relief from pain) in the individual. The areas involved are ventral tegmentum, nucleus accumbens, locus ceruleus, dorsal raphe nucleus and the peri-aqueductal areas.

Psychological Factors

Personality: People with certain personality disorders are more prone to drug dependence than others. These include people with dissocial personality disorder, and traits like sensation seeking and impulsivity.

Learning: According to learning theory both positive and negative reinforcement factors perpetuate the drug habit. Positive reinforcement occurs when the substance rewards the individual with a feeling of well being and relief of pain. The latter occurs when the individual returns to drugs to avoid the distressing withdrawal symptoms.

Social and Environmental Factors

Social attitudes: Social attitudes influence drug taking behavior. Strong disapproval reduces their use. Those substances which are less socially disapproved (e.g. alcohol, and tobacco) are used more freely before moving onto the "hard" drugs (e.g. LSD). The former are therefore sometimes referred to as gateway drugs.

Box 9.2: Clinical Correlates of Drug Use

Acute intoxication: It is a transient condition following drug intake. Symptoms may be different from the primary effects of the drug. Disturbances of sensorium, perception, affect and behavior are common. It is usually dose related and subsides as soon as the drug is stopped and its effects wear off unless complicated by other preexisting conditions, as for example, hepatic damage. Pathological intoxication is an idiosyncratic reaction where even small amounts produce profound intoxication effects.

Withdrawal symptoms: Group of symptoms with a known pattern and which are predictable and time related. They develop on discontinuation of a drug which the individual had been using for a long period, usually in high quantity. Symptoms subside when the withdrawn drug is reintroduced.

Delirium: Withdrawal state may be associated with delirium clinical features of which have been described under organic mental disorders. Though short lived and usually self subsiding delirium may be life-threatening occasionally.

Psychotic disorder: Psychotic disorders may occur concurrently or following use of several psychoactive substances.

Amnestic syndrome: Amnestic syndrome characterized by the disturbances of memory occur following long-term uses of several substances, as for example, alcohol. The clinical features of amnestic syndrome have been described in another chapter.

Residual and chronic effects: Long-term substance use may have several residual effects. They are in the form of flash backs, enduring personality changes, dementia and late onset psychotic symptoms.

Family environment: Alcoholism and drug abuse run in families. Their use by other family members and presence of other forms of psychopathology in the family contribute to the drug taking habit.

Substance availability: It is often the easy accessibility of a particular substance that decides its continued use. This accounts for the higher prevalence of use of such drugs like opiates, stimulants and sedatives among health professionals and continued use of prescription drugs among patients to whom they were prescribed once. Easily and legally available substances (e.g. tobacco preparations and alcohol) are abused more, again for the same reason.

ALCOHOLS

Alcohol unless and otherwise specified refers to ethyl alcohol (ethanol) which is the consumed form of "drink". It is still the most easily available and most abused substance across the world. It may be synthesized but is usually manufactured by fermentation of saccharine liquids by yeast. Cereals, wood or straw may be indirectly fermented and alcohol produced. Dextrose is changed to alcohol by the enzyme zymase of yeast.

Fermentation by yeast is retarded when the alcohol content reaches 15%. Liquors of higher strength are prepared through distillation. Most alcoholic beverages contain between 5% (beer) and 50% (spirits) of alcohol.

Types of Alcohol

Three groups are recognized: (a) malted liquors, (b) wines and (c) spirits. Malted liquors are prepared from cereals by fermentation of the germinating grains. The germinated grain is known as malt and contains maltose which is fermented by yeast. They have an alcohol content between 3 and 7%.

Wines are made by fermentation of the natural sugar of grapes and other fruits. When the whole sugar is fermented the wine is said dry but if the sugar is in excess it is known as sweet. Wines are fortified by adding alcohol as in port and sherry. Champagne is made by charging with carbon dioxide. The alcohol content of wines vary from 5 to 20%.

Spirits are prepared through distillation. Rum is made from molasses and arrack from rice. Gin is distilled over juniper berries.

Box 9.3: Alcohol Content of Some Common Liquors		
Type	*Examples*	*Alcohol content (v/v%)*
Malted liquors	Beer	3 %
	Strong beer	5%
	Extra strong beer	7%
Wines	Table wine	8–10%
	Sherry, Port	15–20%
	Champagne	18–20%
Spirits	Whisky	40%
	Brandy	45–50%
	Rum	50–60%
	Gin	50–60%

Clinical Features

Alcohol brings a sense of warmth, friendliness and increased sociability to the user. Tension is relieved and there is mild euphoria and subjective exhilaration. Inhibitions are lost, talk becomes loquacious. With higher doses signs of intoxication appear.

Intoxication

The person becomes garrulous and argumentative. Euphoria gives way to irritability and hostility or self pity and sadness. There is difficulty in concentrating. Memory lapses, "blackouts" and drowsiness follow. Speech becomes slurred and gait unsteady and coma may ensue. Blackouts are periods during intoxication events of which are not remembered by the patient even though he appears awake and alert. Alcohol may precipitate fits in a person prone to epilepsy. In some people, an idiosyncratic reaction occurs where even small amounts of alcohol lead to excitement and aggressive behavior.

Box 9.4: Blood Alcohol Levels and Behavioural Changes	
Blood alcohol level	Symptoms and observed behavior
10 mg/dl	Sense of warmth, clearing of head
20 mg/dl	Mild dizziness, feeling of well-being, increased sociability
30 mg/dl	Relief of pain and tension, mild euphoria
40 mg/dl	Boisterousness. Talks loudly and excessively
50 mg/dl	Loss of social inhibitions. Takes undue liberty with strangers
70 mg/dl	Movements clumsy; muscular incordination; thinking delayed
100 ml/dl	Drowsy, staggers and falls down. Talks to himself, sings loudly
200 mg/dl	Needs help to walk. Talk garrulously shouts, groans and weeps. Self pity and sadness. Easily angered
300 mg/dl	Stuporous. Breathing slow and stertorous
400 mg/dl	Comatose. May be fatal

Withdrawal

In people who had been taking alcohol for a long time and in excess quantities withdrawal or a reduction in the consumed quantity brings about a host of withdrawal symptoms. The earliest features are the "shakes" - tremors of hands, legs and the trunk which may occur within hours of stopping alcohol. Other symptoms are nausea, vomiting, restlessness and sweating. Perceptual disturbances like illusions and hallucinations are common. Sleep is disturbed and often lacking. Grand mal seizures may occur. Within 24–48 hours delirium tremens (DT) characterized by confusion, disorientation, frightening illusions and hallucinations, tremors and insomnia sets in. Hallucinations are usually visual and the patient is terror stricken. Gross tremors of hands, extreme agitation and restlessness, sweating and tachycardia are also present. Symptoms are worse at night. In its natural course, it lasts for 3 to 4 days and usually subside with a terminal deep prolonged sleep from which the patient wakes up with no memory for the period of delirium. However, delirium tremens has a high risk of mortality in some people requiring intensive care management. Vivid, persistent, visual and auditory hallucinations without delirium may occur in some people.

Long Term Effects

Amnestic Syndrome

Characterised by grossly defective recent memory. Events are recalled immediately but are not retained, and are forgotten a few minutes later. There is no new learning. Confabulation (filling memory gaps with fictions data) is prominent. Other cognitive functions are preserved.

Alcoholic Dementia

Chronic alcoholism causes lasting cognitive impairment, particularly of the frontal lobe function.

Other long-term defects are psychiatric disorders, like alcoholic hallucinosis, delusional disorders (pathological jealousy) impaired psychosexual functions and personality deterioration. Alcoholism has several physical sequelae also.

Physical Effects of Chronic Alcoholism

Liver

Hepatitis, fatty infiltration, cirrhosis and hepatoma.

GI Tract

Neoplasms in the alimentary canal esophageal varices, gastritis, ulcers and malignancy.

Pancreas

Pancreatitis

Heart

Arrhythmias and cardiomyopathy.

Brain and Nervous System

Cerebellar degeneration, dementia, encephalopathy, neuropathy epilepsy.

Reproductive System

Sexual dysfunction testicular atrophy, loss of libido and anovulation.

Fetus

Fetal alcohol syndrome, teratogeny and abortion.

Immunity System

Malnutrition and immunity system suppression.

OPIOIDS

Opioids include opium and its derivations like morphine, heroin and codeine, and the synthetic preparations like pethidine, methadone, buprenorphine (tidigesic), pentazocine (fortwin) and fentanyl. Opium is the air dried milky exudates obtained by incising the unripe capsules of the poppy plant (*Papaver somniferum*). Heroin (diacetylmorphine) colloquially known as brown sugar or smack is prepared from morphine by acetylisation. Codeine is an alkaloid obtained from opium or made artificially from morphine. Pethidine (meperidine hydrochloride) is a synthetic drug not chemically related to morphine. Others are all synthetic opiate preparations.

Patterns of use

Crude opium is smoked, sniffed or eaten by its users where poppy plant is cultivated. Powders of heroin and morphine are dissolved in water and injected directly into veins or subcutaneously (skin popping). Many preparations are available in tablet or powder form and some as injectables illicitly.

Clinical Effects

Opioids produce a dreamy relaxed state of mind with freedom from physical or psychological pains. On long-term use personality changes occur with no motivation or ambition, and neglect of self care.

Withdrawal Effects

Tolerance and dependence develop very rapidly. Withdrawal symptoms are severe and unpleasant, dreaded by the individual. Restlessness, abdominal pain, muscle cramps, nausea, sweating and diarrhea, rhinorrhea, lacrimation and many other symptoms develop 4–8 hours after withdrawal reaching a peak in the next 48–72 hours. They subside afterwards without leaving any permanent ill effects.

CANNABINOIDS

Cannabis indica is the Indian hemp plant locally known as the *Ganja* plant which is cultivated illegally in many hilly regions of Kerala and other states. The main psychoactive constituent of cannabis is THC (tetrahydro cannabinol) which is one of the 60 or more cannabinoids abundant in the flowering tops of the female plant. All parts of the plant contain this in varying amounts. Table 9.2 lists the THC content of various cannabis preparations. Cannabis is known as Marijuana in the west.

Table 9.2: Cannabis preparations		
Preparation	*Plant Parts*	*THC Content*
Bhang	Dried leaves and flowering shoots of plant mixed with poppy seeds and sugar prepared as beverage	1.5%
Ganja	Dried and powderal leaves and inflorescence mixed with tobacco	2%
Hashish (charas)	Resin from the flowering tops of female plants	10–15%
Hashi oil	Fat soluble plant extract	50%

Clinical Features

The preferred way of use is by smoking using cigarettes or special chillums and hookas. Bhang is used as a beverage. The effects vary depending on the person's prevailing mood which is intensified. Peak levels of intoxication occur 15–30 minutes after smoking and lasts for about 4 hours depending on the dose. Behavioral changes will last longer. There is a "high" experience when the time stands still and the individual has a "floating in the air" sensation. Euphoria, heightened introspectivity, ability to appreciate individual senses (e.g. color and sound) more precisely, increased sexual desire and appetite, are all pleasurable effects. Adverse effects are anxiety and fearfulness, perceptual disturbances, derealization and psychotic disturbances. Cannabis can precipitate flash backs of earlier psychotic or painful experiences. Agitation, panic attacks and aggressive outbursts can occur.

Withdrawal symptoms include fear, irritability, disturbed sleep, tremors, tachycardia, increased sweating, muscle pain and occasionally seizures.

SEDATIVES AND HYPNOTICS

This group includes barbiturates and benzodiazepines and some other agents like methaqualone (mandrax), meprobamate, etc. which have high addiction potentials. Clinical effects are similar to those of alcohol intoxication along with mild euphoria and a pleasant soothing drowsiness are noted by the user. Intoxication leads to confusion drowsiness and ataxia. Speech is slurred. Coma may ensue.

Withdrawal symptoms are characterized by restlessness, irritability, insomnia and excitement. Tachycardia, sweating, tremors, nausea and vomiting are other features. There may be perceptual disturbances and withdrawal seizures may occur.

COCAINE

Cocaine is derived from the leaves of coca plant (erythrocylon coca) which is indigenous to South America. Its leaves are chewed by natives to relieve fatigue and suppress hunger. Cocaine hydrochloride is a white crystalline powder. The substance is administered through different routes — chewing, sniffing, smoking and injecting. "Crack" cocaine is a prepackaged form.

Clinically cocaine increases mental alertness, and produces increased energy and euphoria. Social disinhibition, sexual arousal, heightened self-esteem which on intoxication leads to psychomotor agitation, tachycardia, visual and tactile hallucinations ("Cocaine bug") and aggressive behavior. Frank delirium may occur with continuous use. A clinical picture resembling delusional disorder is seen.

Withdrawal symptoms are heralded by dysphagia or "the crash". Depression, anhedonia, insomnia, anxiety, irritability and intense cocaine craving follow. There are vivid and unpleasant dreams. There may be suicidal thoughts. On continued abstinence craving becomes lesser and a desire to sleep supercedes. Craving and hypersomnia follows with relief of all symptoms.

AMPHETAMINES

Amphetamines with other related substances like methyl-phenidate, and phenmetrazine belong to the stimulant group of drugs. Caffeine is also included in this group in ICD-10.

Amphetamine is a synthetic substance and is popularly called as the "speed" or "Pep pill". It is taken orally, but can be smoked or injected. Taken orally it heightens mood and keeps the individual wakeful and alert. Euphoria and overactivity are present. It suppresses hunger. Adverse effects on intoxication are insomnia, headache and irritability along with visual hallucinations. It precipitates psychosis with persecutory delusions similar to paranoid schizophrenia.

Withdrawal symptoms include dysphoria, fatigue, vivid and unpleasant dreams and hypersomnia. Craving is present.

Other substances also have similar properties and actions. Psychosis is rare. Caffeine gives mental alertness, and mild euphoria, withdrawal of which leads to headache, drowsiness, fatigue and impaired concentration on psychomotor activities.

HALLUCINOGENS

Hallucinogens are psychoactive substances which bring about perceptual disturbances along with concurrent mood changes. Some hallucinogens are naturally occurring like psilocybin (extracted from species of mushrooms), mescaline (from the cactus, peyote) hemaline and ibogaine (some species of shrubs) and LSD (ergot alkaloids). Ergot is the compact mycelium of a fungus (claviceps) which grows in the ovary of Rye. LSD can be synthesized as also MDA (methylene dioxy amphetamine) and MDMA (methylene dioxy meth-amphetamine). LSD is an extremely potent drug and produces effects in doses as small as 30 micrograms.

Effects of hallucinogens vary depending on the individual and setting. Intense perceptual changes in time, space and body image occur. The person is alert to the changes which he is able to narrate. Time stands still rich with pleasurable events. Illusions and hallucinations, primarily visual but in other modalities also occur, sometimes in altered sense modalities. Thus the subject may report of feeling colors and seeing sounds (synesthesia). Intense emotional and mystic experiences are common (e.g. own body merging with the surroundings; feeling togetherness with the world). Physical signs of intoxication are increased heart rate, sweating, piloerection and dilatation of pupils. Experiences may not always be pleasant ("bad trips") but may be painful and terrifying during which time there are risks of suicide.

Withdrawal effects include craving, anergia, depression and physical distress.

TOBACCO

The chief active constituent of tobacco is nicotine which gives a soothing effect for chronic users, particularly after deprivation. This accounts for the first cigarette of the day being more enjoyable. Nicotine helps to concentrate better. Toxic effects are nausea, abdominal pain, salivation, headache, cold sweat and amblyopia.

Withdrawal effects are dysphoria, irritability, restlessness and poor concentration.

VOLATILE SOLVENTS

Inhaling volatile solvents is a form of drug abuse and involves such diverse substances like petrol, spray paints, varnishes, glues, lighter fluids, nail polish and a variety of cleansing fluids. They are inhaled directly from the tins or bottles or by smelling rags soaked in the fluid. Sometimes plastic bags containing the substance are applied to the mouth for inhaling or the substances are directly sprayed into the mouth. Clinical effects include grandiosity, exhilaration and perceptual changes. Ataxia, blurring of vision, psychosis and drowsiness leading to coma are the common adverse effects. Those who resort to inhalant abuse often indulge in disruptive antisocial behavior after getting intoxicated. Deaths have occurred following inhalant intoxication.

GENERAL PRINCIPLES OF TREATMENT

The aim of treatment is to make the individual, free from drugs and the resulting complications. The methods and agents used depend on the drug and the individual. The treatment program involves several steps:

    i. Early identification

    ii. Motivating the individual to give up the habit

    iii. Withdrawal of the substance totally or partially

    iv. Treating the complications and associated conditions

    v. Preventing relapses

    vi. Rehabilitation

Early Identification

Early identification is needed to prevent drug use from getting established and to stall development of dependence. Management is easier in nondependent cases.

Enhancing Motivation

Enhancing motivation is valuable when the drug user is aware of his problems but is not sure whether he can overcome them. Persuasion and not a dogmatic enforcement of the therapist's views is to be resorted to. Instead of arguments the patient should be helped to find out himself the ways of overcoming the habit and the risks in continuing the drug.

Drug Withdrawal

Withdrawal of the substance (detoxification) involves different strategies like (a) gradually taper off the dose so as not cause undue distress to the patient and ultimately take off the drug totally, (b) if total withdrawal is not possible bring it down to a considerably low and safe level, (c) use substitute drugs, (d) using drugs which affects withdrawal mechanisms (as for example, clonidine in opioid withdrawal) and e. symptomatic measures. In severely dependent cases a controlled use of the substance will be more feasible than total abstinence.

Management of Consequences and Complications

Intravenous use of drugs often has devastating consequences such as thrombosis of veins, local and systemic infections due to the unsterile apparatus. Complications, both physical and psychiatric are often encountered as a result of prolonged drug use or due to intoxication. These should be attended to preventing relapses.

Measures to prevent relapses include adopting alternate methods of coping, change of environment and use of pharmacological agents (e.g. anti-craving agents, disulfiram in alcohol). Nonpharmacological methods include participation in self help groups like A.A, Al-anon, etc.

Rehabilitation

For successful rehabilitation the patient should be weaned away from the drug subculture and encouraged to make new social contacts. He should be engaged in gainful activities in a therapeutic community or in other sheltered surroundings before seeking opportunities independently in the wider social setting.

10

Psychiatry and Medicine

It is a well known fact that psychological factors affect physical (i.e. organic) medical conditions. Genesis, course, response to treatment and the outcome of a physical disease is greatly influenced by emotional factors. Such conditions or disorders where emotional factors play a decisive role were once known as psychophysiological disorders. The term was replaced by "psychosomatic disorders" in 1918 by Heinroth who coined that term. Franz Alexander, a prominent advocate of the psychosomatic theory proposed that seven disorders were psychosomatic—bronchial asthma, rheumatoid arthritis, ulcerative colitis, essential hypertension, neurodermatitis, thyrotoxicosis and peptic ulcer. He differentiated hysterical conversion reactions (dissociation disorders) from "organ neuroses" by pointing out that psychosomatic disorders occurred only in organs innervated by autonomic nervous system. They do not have a symbolic meaning and they are the end results of chronic physiological malfunctioning.

Psychosomatic disorders were designated as psychophysiologic disorders in 1952 by the American Psychiatric Association and the term was used in the DSM-II classification (1968) with 10 categories (skin, musculoskeletal, respiratory, cardiovascular, lymphatic, gastrointestinal, genitourinary, endocrine, organs of special sense and others). In the next edition (DSM-III, 1980) the terminology was again changed and a category named "Psychological Factors Affecting Physical Conditions (PFAPC)" was introduced. This is retained in the latest revision (DSM-IV, 1994) also after an extensive evaluation of the clinical conditions in the category. In ICD-10 these disorders are listed under "psychological and behavioral factors associated with disorders or diseases classified elsewhere (F54) where they are specified by using two codes — F54 and the additional code of the disorder (as for example, Bronchial asthma F54 plus 145. X).

More and more diseases or disorders are included in the psychosomatic rubric with the discovery of their psycho-biological genesis and predisposition. Some of them are listed in Table 10.1. Genetic vulnerability and the patient's physical condition constitute the biological factors. Personality and specific emotional conflicts are the psychological factors. Social factors are the life events and stresses. Personality and the biological factors act as the predisposing factors making the individual vulnerable to the illness. The time at which the illness is precipitated is often decided by the conflicts and stresses of that period.

PSYCHOLOGICAL REACTION TO ILLNESS

Every individual reacts emotionally to his illness. The type of reaction and its intensity and duration vary widely depending on several factors. The most common reaction patterns are the following:

Table 10.1: Some common "psychosomatic" disorders	
Respiratory disorders	Bronchial asthma, vasomotor rhinitis, COPD (chronic obstructive pulmonary disease)
Gastrointestinal disorders	Irritable bowel syndrome, peptic ulcer, obesity, inflammatory bowel diseases, anorexia nervosa
Cardiovascular disorders	Essential hypertension, coronary artery disease
Skin disorders	Psoriasis, eczema, pruritis, hyper-hydrosis, urticaria
Musculoskeletal disorders	Rheumatoid arthritis
Endocrine disorders	Diabetes mellitus, hyperthyroidism, hypothyroidism, Cushing's syndrome
Immunity disorders	Allergic disorders, autoimmune disorders
Psychosexual disorders	Premature ejaculation, frigidity, dys-pareunia, impotence
Psychogenic pain	Headache, myalgias

a. **Anxiety:** The earliest and the commonest reaction to illness is anxiety. Anxiety is universal and may precede the actual diagnosis of the main illness being evident even when some of its symptoms are manifest. The threat of an impending serious illness and its repercussions on himself and his family are the precipitants of anxiety. Anxiety sometimes may be the heralding symptom of an oncoming illness. It may manifest as a feeling of apprehensive restlessness, insomnia, palpitations and other autonomic disturbances. The intensity also may vary from a mild feeling of anxiety to panic needing special management strategies from a calm assurance to medication.

b. **Depression:** Like anxiety depression also may be a heralding symptom of the main illness. Depression is common among patients with chronic illnesses particularly if they lead to permanent invalidity. Whether threat is genuine or imagined, diseases perceived as life threatening, produce intense depression with suicidal risk to the patient. When the coping abilities are minimal or when they are depleted a major depressive episode may be precipitated indistinguishable from a depressive disorder. Hopelessness and helplessness, tearfulness, fatigue, loss of energy, insomnia and other symptoms of clinical depression are encountered in various degrees.

c. **Denial:** Denial of the illness is also a common emotional reaction. As a defense mechanism it averts anxiety but when anxiety is severe the mechanism fails. Denial is manifested as minimizing the severity of symptoms, by wearing a smiling carefree countenance even when there is obvious disparity between the patient's real condition and how it is reported. Denial is common among those who are drug dependent in spite of them having severe physical complications.

d. **Regression:** Regression to a passive dependent state is another type of reaction, particularly adopted by people with a dependent personality. He frees himself from all responsibilities of self care and wants others to wait and care for him. Hospitalization and bed rest encourage regression and in a susceptible patient it leads him to seek secondary gains like sympathy, attention and, even monetary help.

FACTORS AFFECTING THE EMOTIONAL RESPONSE

A variety of factors influence the nature of emotional response. These include the personality of the patient (as for example, those with a dependent personality adopt a "help me" attitude, severity of illness (as for example, life-threatening illnesses leads to severe anxiety and depression), family and social support, and hospital environment (aggravation of anxiety and insecurity feelings mooted by a non-friendly environment.

PSYCHIATRY AND PHYSICAL DISORDERS

Very often a psychiatric disorder coexists with a physical disorder. Apart from such independent coexistence of the two disorders there are other types of association between them — namely:

1. Psychological factors causing physical disorders.
2. Psychiatric disorders presenting as a physical disorder.
3. Physical disorders producing psychiatric symptoms.

Psychological Factors Causing Physical Disorders

Mention was made earlier, in the beginning of the chapter about disorders where psychological factors are the decisive factors in the genesis or aggravation. The psychophysiological or psychosomatic disorders (Table 10.1) belong to this group. However, a wider etiology where biological, psychological and social factors are all important by their presence and mutual interaction was proposed by later workers, a view which is currently held.

Psychiatric Disorders Pesenting with Physical Symptoms

Disorders presenting with physical symptoms, where there is no organic pathology to account for the symptoms belong to this group. Examples are a group of disorders classified as somatoform disorders. In ICD-10 somatoform disorders (F45) are listed as a category in the same block containing neurotic and stress related disorders (F 40–48). They are characterized by repeated presentation of physical symptoms suggesting a general medical condition. However, the symptoms have no organic basis as seen by the negative findings on repeated investigations. Also the distress caused is out of proportion to the extent of symptoms. Significant impairment in social and occupational areas of functioning is present. There may be strong evidence for psychogenesis, though this is denied by the patient. Somatoform disorders differ from factitious disorder and malingering in that they are not feigned or intentionally produced, i.e. not under voluntary control. They differ from PFAPC (psychological factors affecting physical condition) in that there is no diagnosable physical condition to account for the symptoms.

    a. Somatization disorder

    b. Hypochondriacal disorder

    c. Somatoform autonomic function

    d. Persistent somatoform pain disorders.

a. Somatization Disorder

This is characterized by the presence of recurrent multiple symptoms of long duration for which medical treatment is resorted. The symptoms cause significant impairment in social functioning. Any part of the body may be affected but the commonest are those related to gastrointestinal (pain, dyspepsia, belching, nausea and diarrhea), reproductive (erectile dysfunction, irregular menstrual periods, etc.) and neurological (ataxia, weakness, headache, seizures, etc.) systems. Many undergo surgery and repeated medical investigations and take medicines in excessive quantities to the point of dependence. The disorder run a chronic course with fluctuations in intensity.

b. Hypochondriacal disorder

Hypochondriacal disorder (hypochondriasis) is characterized by the patient's preoccupation with fear of having a serious, not yet detected disease. To detect the underlying illness he requests for further investigations. Hypochondriasis differs from somatization disorder in two aspects. In somatization disorder the patient is distressed by his symptoms which he requests to be removed. In hypochondriacal disorder the patient is morbidly afraid of having a serious illness and requests for more and more investigations to detect it. He assumes that an illness is present from the various signs and physical symptoms, of which he is not primarily bothered. The patient with somatization disorder is morbidly concerned of his symptoms and his primary concern is the symptom removal. Secondly, the hypochondriacal patient is afraid to take tablets because of the supposed adverse effects unlike the patient with somatization disorder who indiscriminately uses medicines. Disease conviction and disease phobia characterize hypochondriacal disorders — though the conviction is not of a delusional proportion. He can acknowledge the possibility that he may not have the feared illness. However no assurance or negative investigation findings allay his fears. Reports of another person having the feared illness of even casual remarks about his illness make him unduly perturbed.

c. Somatoform Autonomic Dysfunction

Any organ or system with autonomic innervation may be affected in somatoform autonomic dysfunctions. The presenting symptoms include palpitations, "missed beats" and chest pain (cardiovascular system), hyperventilation and breathlessness (respiratory system), diarrhea and bloating (gastrointestinal system). The organ or system shows no structural or functional abnormality.

d. Somatoform Pain Disorder

Persistent and severe pain which is not explainable physically and which occurs in association with emotional stress is the essential feature of somatoform pain disorder.

Physical Disorders with Psychiatric Sequelae

Many physical disorders have their psychiatric sequelae which are either a direct effect of the disease or the effects of drugs used to treat it or an indirect one where the illness acts as a stressor on the organism. Some medical conditions which present with psychiatric symptoms are listed in Table 10.2.

Table 10.2: Some physical illnesses with psychiatric symptoms

Disease	Psychiatric symptoms
Essential hypertension	Fatigue, anxiety, depression
Myocardial infarction	Depression
Bronchial asthma	Irritability, depression
Pellagra, beriberi	Fatigue, depression, paranoid ideas, delirium, depression, irritability, apathy, confusion, delirium
Pernicious anemia (B_{12} deficiency)	Fatigue, malaise, depression, irritability
Myxedema	Lethargy, loss of interest, irritability, depression, paranoid ideas
Thyrotoxicosis	Anxiety
Cushing's syndrome	Acute anxiety, depression, paranoid delusions
Addison's disease	Apathy, depression, paranoid ideas
Diabetes mellitus	Lethargy, depression
Hypoglycemia	Anxiety, dread, confusion, delusions, hallucinations
Viral fevers	Depression
Enteric fever	Clouding of consciousness, euphoria or depression
Pulmonary TB	Malaise, fatigue, euphoria
HIV infection	Anxiety, depression
Anoxia	Anxiety, hallucinations, confusion
Porphyria	Anxiety, mood swings
Hepatic failure	Euphoria or depression, emotional lability and incontinence, delirium
Uremia	Delirium, psychosis
Cardiac failure	Emotional lability, delirium

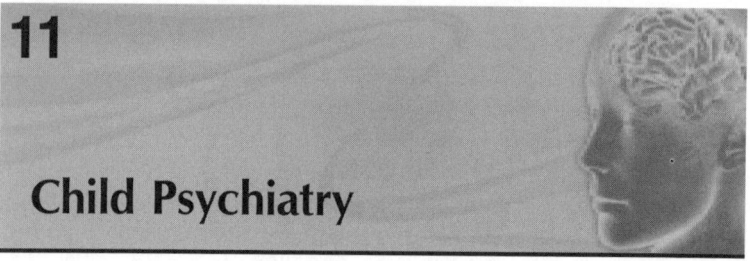

11

Child Psychiatry

Child psychiatry evolved as a major subspeciality and as an independent discipline only some fifty years ago inspired by the recognition that children are not miniature adults. There are certain disorders which occur exclusively in childhood and there are several others whose genesis can be traced to the early developmental period.

CLASSIFICATION

According to the International Classification (ICD–10) psychiatric disorders of childhood are grouped as follows:

I. Disorders of psychological development
  a. Specific developmental disorders of speech and language
  b. Specific developmental disorders of scholastic skills
  c. Specific developmental disorders of motor functions
  d. Pervasive developmental disorders

II. Behavioral and emotional disorders with onset usually occurring in childhood and adolescence
  a. Hyperkinetic disorders
  b. Conduct disorders
  c. Emotional disorders with onset specific to childhood
  d. Disorders of social functioning with onset specific to childhood and adolescence
  e. Other disorders

I. DISORDERS OF PSYCHOLOGICAL DEVELOPMENT

This group includes disorders characterized by a delay in maturation or development of various functions. The functions affected are speech and language, scholastic skills like reading, writing and arithmetic and motor functions. They are invariably noted during infancy and childhood and are carried into adult life, in a less intense manner steadily without remissions or relapses.

The group also includes disorders where the defect is not a delay but a deviance or impairment of functioning (e.g. autism). In almost all of them (whether delay or deviance) the defect is manifest at the very beginning without a normal phase intervening but in a few a short normal phase of development may be seen before the defects become clinically evident.

It is emphasized that such disorders are a resultant of maturational delay and not attributed to general retardation, environmental deprivation like lack of opportunities and also not secondary to a prevailing organic pathology or mental illness.

    a. **Speech and language:** Developmental disorders of speech and language are also known as communication disorders. Disorders of speech present as defects of articulation. Proper articulation of most sounds is achieved normally by the age of seven. When articulation is defective it results in mispronunciations, lalling or lisping. In lalling consonants r and 1 are pronounced imprecisely (as for example, "broken reed" is pronounced as "bwoken weed"). In lisping sibilants (s, z, th, ch) are mispronounced (as for example's is substituted with th — "sweet" as thweet").
Language disorder may be receptive or expressive. In the former there is failure in understanding language (comprehension) and the child does not respond to familiar names. In expressive language disorder comprehension is normal but expression is defective. It is seen as difficulty in selecting proper words or as grammatical errors. Vocabulary is also limited.

    b. **Scholastic skills:** Scholastic skills include those of reading, writing and mathematics (the three "r"s—reading, riting and 'rthmetic). Symptoms of reading disorder are inaccurate word recognition, slowness and errors of oral reading and poor comprehension of written text, words or morphemes (meaningful parts of the word) are misread—distorted, omitted or substituted. Words are re-read, revised and rechecked which makes reading slow particularly when the words are unfamiliar. This occurs both in oral and silent reading. Words are sometimes reversed ("backward reading"). Comprehension is also affected.

Disorders of written expression present as impaired ability to compose written text. Sentences are poorly formed and there are errors in spelling punctuation, grammar and syntax. Spelling errors are the commonest (e.g. offen for often; caim for came, etc.) There may be reversal as dog for god. Excessively poor handwriting may be indicative of a writing disorder.

Arithmetic skill (mathematics) disorder usually affects the basic functions like addition, subtraction, etc. and not the complex ones. Symbols and mathematical signs are not recognized (perceptual symptoms) and there are operational errors, as in counting, following sequential steps, etc. Some show difficulty in coding verbal problems into mathematical symbols. Others have difficulty in forming concepts, as for example, first and last, more or less, before and after, etc. Yet others exhibit symptoms resembling attentional deficits like inaccurate copying of digits and symbols, omitting or misplacing (for example, decimal points) them, etc. but they are not due to carelessness but are due to lack of understanding.

c. **Motor skills:** Disorders of motor functions are characterized by an impairment of motor coordination in the absence of neurological deficits. There is delay in achieving motor milestones (crawling, sitting, walking, etc.) and the movements are clumsy and not precise. Fine (writing, sewing, tying shoe lace) and gross (walking, running, etc.) motor coordination skills are affected. Specific manifestations may vary from one child to another and all functions are not affected together in a uniform manner. Often they suffer from other developmental or learning difficulties. There may be associated peer group problems, often secondary to the motor function defects. Many coordination disorders improve over time and show no further deterioration, though they are still inferior to normal controls even years later.

d. **Pervasive developmental disorders:**

Autism

Autistic disorder or infantile autism as Kanner named it in 1943 is a pervasive developmental disorder characterized by widespread (hence called pervasive) and severe disturbances in several areas of functioning. The disorder manifests itself within the first five years of life and may be associated with chromosomal anomalies and metabolic disorders like cerebral lipidoses. One in a thousand children is the estimated prevalence rate in the general population. The disorder is up to four times more common in boys than girls.

Etiology

Unknown but genetic influence (50 times more common among twins than in general population), chromosomal abnormalities and organic brain disorders have been postulated as possible causes.

Clinical Features

Three main features were listed by Kanner which are still used as diagnostic:

a. **Abnormalities in social interactions:** This was viewed by Kanner as the core deficit. There is a lack of social reciprocation as seen by not raising hands in readiness for being picked up or being passive during cuddling. They avoid eye contact. There is no social play with other children. They are equally unresponsive to parents or strangers and show little anxiety when left in unfamiliar surroundings.

b. **Abnormalities of communication:** There is usually a delay in development of language. Echolalia (repeating the same words spoken to him), articulation difficulties and pronominal reversal (referring to self as "you" and to others as "I") are common.

c. **Stereotyped behavior:** These include activities like jumping up and down, hand flapping and finger wriggling, rocking movements of body, spinning and moving the extended fingers in front of their eyes. Their play is rigid and restricted like rolling bottles or filtering sand through fingers. Autistic children insist on sameness in food, dress and behavior and resist changes in their environment. They want the same toys, the same dress, the same food and the same bowls.

Other features include hypersensitivity to sounds, food faddism, mood disturbances like self smiling, laughing and crying for no apparent reason. Some children inflict self injury by biting their own fingers or banging their head on the wall. Many autistic children have associated seizure disorder. EEG shows several abnormalities.

Treatment

Special schooling and residential schooling may be needed, the latter when the symptoms are severe and the child is unmanageable at home. Individual psychotherapy and behavior modification procedures are useful. Drugs are necessary when target symptoms like aggression, self injury and hyperactivity are present. Lithium, amphetamine, haloperidol, pimozide and clonidine have been tried with variable success. Drugs are withdrawn periodically (once in 3–6 months) to assess improvement and necessity of continuing treatment.

Course and Prognosis

Autistic disorder continues as a lifelong disability though over the course of time some improvement is achieved in language functions and social relations. However, many children are unable to lead an independent existence.

II. EMOTIONAL AND BEHAVIOR DISORDERS OF CHILDHOOD

This is a group of miscellaneous disorders, onset of which is usually traceable to childhood and adolescence. Some of them (e.g. emotional disorders) which specifically occur in childhood and adolescence differ from similar disorders seen in adults both in their presentation and etiology. Others, however, have no such clear distinction and are identical in their origin, pathology and clinical presentation.

Hyperkinetic Disorders

Hyperkinetic disorders are characterized by restlessness and overactivity, impulsiveness and impaired attention. Such behavior occurs both at home and in school and pervades all activities of the child. The symptoms appear before school age and continue becoming milder as the child grows older. The disorder is more frequent among boys than girls.

Because of the impaired attention and lack of persistence the child shifts from one task to another leaving each job unfinished. Overactivity shows as extreme restlessness, the child jumping up and running around aimlessly. Because of recklessness and impulsiveness the child is prone to accidents. Associated abnormalities are aggressiveness, temper tantrums and insubordination.

Genetic and social factors are implied in the etiology of the disorder.

Stimulant drugs like amphetamine and methylphenidate have been tried in hyperkinetic disorders. In a good percentage of children they help to improve attention deficits, at least on a short-term basis. Treatment may be needed for several months or even years. Their long-term benefits are uncertain. Other drugs which have been found useful are antidepressants (e.g. imipramine) and neuroleptics (e.g. haloperidol). Behavior therapy and remedial teaching are also helpful.

Conduct Disorders

These are persistent (and not isolated) dissocial (antisocial) behavior which includes telling lies, defiance, stealing, truancy, destruction of property and aggression and cruelty to people and animals. Such behavior occurs either at home or school and may be associated with alcohol and drug abuse. In adolescents sexual promiscuity or reckless sexual practices may lead to teenage pregnancy and other complications.

Genetic and environmental factors are believed to be causative. Children with epilepsy and brain damage are more susceptible to conduct disorder. They run a prolonged course and may be carried to adulthood as dissocial personality disorder.

Behavioral modes of treatment have been tried along with anger management training. Among drugs methylphenidate and amphetamine decrease aggression. Other agents which have anti-aggressive properties are lithium, carbamazepine and haloperidol. Residential care may be needed when unmanageable at home.

Emotional Disorders

According to the International Classification (ICD-10) emotional disorders which occur specifically during childhood and adolescence are differentiated from adult neurotic disorders in several respects. Emotional disorders of childhood are often exaggerations of normal developmental patterns. Children and adolescents often outgrow them by adulthood. Adults who have these symptoms mostly develop them during adult life without evincing their presence in their childhood years.

The main emotional disorders of childhood are separation anxiety, phobic anxiety disorder, social anxiety disorder and sibling rivalry disorder. Separation anxiety disorder is characterized by excessive and unrealistic anxiety during periods of separation from parents. It shows as multiple somatic complaints (headache, etc.) crying and tantrums. The child may refuse to attend school due to separation anxiety.

Phobias are common in children but they outgrow them by early teens. In phobic anxiety disorder the phobias persist in an exaggerated manner even beyond. In social anxiety disorder the children are markedly anxious in the presence of unfamiliar people and avoid all forms of social contacts with them. Sibling rivalry is shown as jealousy and competition against a younger sibling which persist and find expression through hostile interactions and physical trauma.

Obsessive compulsive disorders are rare in children even though children indulge in many repetitive and ritualistic behavior-like avoiding cracks on the pavement while walking, arranging one's things in a fixed pattern, etc.

In addition to the above many emotional disorders which are seen in adults (e.g. mood disorders) occur in children also.

Disorders of Social Functioning

This category refers to some abnormalities in social functioning noted during childhood. They differ from pervasive developmental disorders in their absence of a constitutional defect and in that they do not pervade all areas of the child's functioning. Elective mutism is an example where the child is "normal" at home or while among close friends but is mute at school or among strangers.

Other Behavior Disorders

They constitute an array of heterogeneous disorders which are seen in children and adolescents.

a. *Tic disorders:* Tics are abrupt, non-purposive stereotyped, repetitive movements involving circumscribed muscle groups. Motor tics involve contraction of a muscle group. Those involving face cause such acts like blinking, sniffing, grimacing, tongue darting, lip smacking, etc. Those involving the upper arms result in such acts like shrugging the shoulders. Those affecting the diaphragm produce grunting or barking sounds.

Compulsive coughing, throat clearing, spitting, etc. are other examples. The child has an urge to carry out the act often against his will to control them. Tics are common in childhood and vary in their intensity. They are more common in boys.

Gilles de la tourette's syndrome (GTS)

This is a complex neurological disorder characterized by multiple tics, vocalization like corprolalia (uttering obscene words), palilalia (pathological repetitions of the same syllables) and echolalia (repetition of words which the child hears from people around). The child makes coughing, grunting or barking sounds, grunts his teeth and makes skipping or jumping movements. The disorder starts in pre-pubertal age and has a benign course. It disappears during sleep but is exaggerated during emotional turmoil. Haloperidol and pimozide are effective in controlling the symptoms. The disorder occurs more commonly in boys than girls.

b. *Enuresis* is involuntary voiding of urine persisting even beyond 5 years of age and may be diurnal or nocturnal, nocturnal being more common. Organic causes are to be ruled out. Toilet training and restricting fluids at night are advocated. Behavior therapy using the "bell and pad" apparatus is helpful. The bell rings when the pad gets wet on voiding and wakes up the child. Drugs like imipramine are also of value.

c. *Encopresis* is involuntary fecal soiling which persists after the age of 5 years or which occurs after normal bowel control is achieved. Organic causes like a ganglionic megacolon and spina bifida are to be ruled out.

d. *Feeding disorders* are persistent disturbances of eating in the form of refusal or food fads. Pica is eating non-nutritive substances like mud, hair, paper, etc.

e. *Stammering* is a disturbance of rhythm and fluency of speech where speech is hesitated spasmodic and interrupted. *Stuttering* is also a form of faltered speech characterized by repetitions or prolongations of sounds and syllables. *Cluttering* is rapid and disrhythmic flow of words characterized by alternating pauses and bursts of speech.

MENTAL RETARDATION

Mental retardation is defined as a state of arrested or incomplete development of intellectual functions, manifested as impairment of cognitive, language and adaptive functions seen at the time of birth or early developmental years. In the past several terms were used to denote the condition, like mental subnormality, feeble mindedness, mental handicap, mental deficiency, etc.

PREVALENCE

The prevalence rate varies depending on the severity and criteria used to measure retardation. The overall prevalence is estimated as 10–20 per thousand for the whole population. There are several grades of mental retardation, which are— mild, moderate, severe and profound (see below) and their overall rates vary from 1.7% (mild) to 0.02% (profound) of the total population. With better antenatal, perinatal and neonatal care the incidence of mental retardation has substantially reduced over the years.

Classification

According to the International Classification mental retardation is classified into four grades depending on the intelligence test scores or IQ (intelligence quotient — see below) obtained by administration of standard intelligence tests. A test score of 100 or around indicates normal intelligence. Mental retardation is said to exist when the scores are less then 70. The cutting points for the four grades of retardation according to ICD-10 are shown below:

Mild mental retardation	IQ	50–69
Moderate	IQ	35–49
Severe	IQ	20–34
Profound	IQ	below 20

Box 11.1: Measuring Intelligence

In 1904 Binet, a French psychologist was assigned the task of identifying school children who did not benefit from the usual teaching methods because of their low intelligence. Along with Simon, one of his colleagues he developed a series of tests of graded difficulty in an age appropriated manner so that most children of a particular age (say, 5 years) could accomplish the tests designed for that age group. Children below that age group (say, 4 years) failed to do them and those of a higher age group (say, 6 years) could do them with no difficulty. The tests were administered to a large population of children and test items were selected based on these findings. A five-year-old child who could do the tests appropriated to that age was considered normal, i.e., of normal intelligence. If he could do the tests set for a higher age level (say, 6-year-old) he was considered superior. Like wise he was considered inferior if he could not do the five year level tests and was able to do the four year level tests only. An intelligent quotient (IQ) was than devised as a useful indicator of the intellectual level.

$$\text{Intelligent Quotient (IQ)} = \frac{\text{Mental Age (MA)} \times 100}{\text{Chronological Age (CA)}}$$

where the mental age denotes the age level of the tests and chronological age the biological age of the child. Several intelligence tests were subsequently developed offering universal applicability by eliminating cultural bias of the items.

Intelligence and its Distribution

Intelligence was once conceptualized as a fixed trait, a trait which a person is born with and which never changes. Even though it is highly heritable, as demonstrated by twin studies it is also "malleable" meaning that it can be modified by such factors as socioeconomic and cultural enrichment and education. The IQ scores across different cultures and countries of the world however represent only one part of the intelligence and does not reveal the capacity for adaptive behavior which is also a measure of intelligence.

When IQ scores are plotted against population, a bell-shaped curve is obtained statistically described as a "normal distribution". About two-thirds of the population have IQ scores falling between 85 and 115. About 16% have IQ scores ranging from 85 to 70 and 115 to 130 at either ends and some 2% below 70 or above 130 at the tapering ends of the curve (Fig. 11.1).

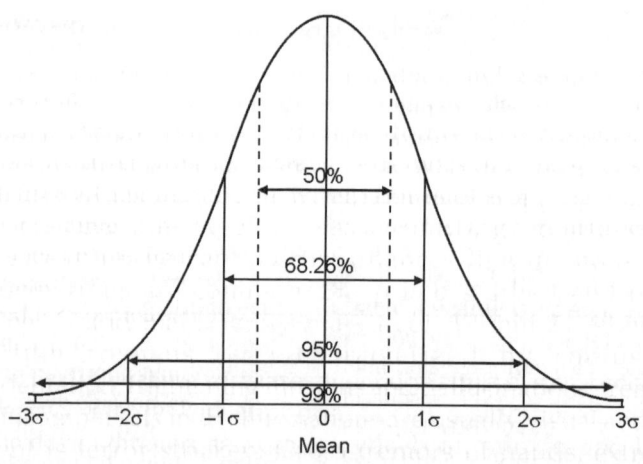

Fig. 11.1: Distribution of intelligence. The figure shows the "normal" bell shaped frequency curve. The scores concentrate in and around the center (mean) and taper out to the two tail ends. 68% of the distribution scores lie between +1 SD and −1 SD (standard deviation, a measure of variability). 95% lie between +2 and −2 SD and 99% between +3 and −3 SD (see text)

ETIOLOGY

Mental retardation has multiple causes—both organic and environmental. In the more severe forms of retardation organic causes predominate.

The etiological factors can be conveniently grouped into prenatal, perinatal and postnatal factors. More than one factor may operate at any instance with additive effects.

Prenatal Factors

The important prenatal factors are genetic and chromosomal aberrations, prematurity, congenital anomalies, maternal factors and complications of pregnancy.

Box 11.2: Down Syndrome

Named after Down, an English physician of the 19th century it is the commonest genetic cause of learning disability (mental retardation). In the general population, it has a frequency of one in 700 live births but with advancing age of the mother it's frequency rises – some 20 times more frequent in mother's over 45 years of age than those who are less than 30.

The condition is due to a chromosomal aberration and in most cases (95% of all cases) it relates to the 21st pair by having an additional chromosome (Trisomy-21). More than a 100 signs (stigmata) have been described for the condition. The commonest are slanting palpebral fissures (88%), hyperextensible joints (88%), flabby hands (84%), brachy cephalic skull with flat occiput (80%), ear anomalies (80%), high arched palate (75%) and irregular alignment of teeth (75%). Often there are other congenital defects and many of the affected children have only a single palmar transverse crease instead of the usual two.

The severity of mental retardation varies from moderate to severe degree though they give an impression of higher mental capacity. Life expectancy used to be around 12 years but with advanced medical facilities many view for more than 50 years.

Retardation due to genetic factors is seen in epiloia (tuberous sclerosis), neurofibromatosis and the various inborn errors of metabolism. The former two have an autosomal dominant inheritance whereas most of the errors of metabolism have a recessive inheritance. Some inborn metabolic disorders associated with mental retardation are: phenylketonuria (PKU, homocystinuria and Hartnup disease (errors of amino acid metabolism), Tay-Sachs disease, Gaucher's disease and

Niemann-Pick disease (errors of lipid metabolism); galacto-semia, glycogen storage diseases and fructose tolerance disease (errors of carbohydrate metabolism). Down syndrome and cat cry syndromes are examples of autosomal chromosomal aberrations. Klinefelter's syndrome (XXY) and Turner's syndrome (X0) are sex linked chromosomal aberrations.

Box 11.3: Phenylketonuria (PKU)

PKU is a well studied metabolic disorder causing mental retardation. The metabolism of phenylalanine, an essential amino acid is deranged due to the absence of a liver enzyme phenyl alanine hydroxylase. This enzyme is needed to convert phenylalanine to tyrosine. Its absence leads to accumulation of phenylalanine in the blood and retards myelination of nerve tissues leading to MR. Tyrosine is needed to synthesize serotonin an important neuro humor which also is diminished due to lack of tyrosine.

PKU affects one person in 15000 of general population and accounts for 1% of all mentally retarded children. The mental retardation is of the severe degree. Microcephaly, eczema, hyperactivity and convulsions are features.

PKU is a preventable disease. Treatment is dietary restriction of phenyl-alanine. The dietary regimen should continue till about 6 years of age–by which time brain differentiation is complete. Women who had PKU are at high risk for bearing children with PKU and in them dietary restriction should start prior to conception and continue till delivery is over.

Congenital anomalies like neural tube defects, microcephaly, macrocephaly and porencephaly (cystic formation in the cerebral hemispheres) also account for mental retardation. Maternal infections during pregnancy, particularly in the first trimester (e.g. rubella, syphilis, toxoplasmosis), intoxications (e.g. alcohol), trauma (hypoxia, radiation) and complications of pregnancy (e.g. placenta previa, maternal diseases, malnutrition) also have deleterious effects in the child resulting in mental retardation.

Perinatal Factors

Abnormal fetal presentations resulting in prolonged labor and birth injuries (mechanical as from application of forceps, or due to anoxia) are the main perinatal factors. Anoxia may be due to obstruction by mucus plugs inside the trachea, or due to medicines causing respiratory depression. Neonatal jaundice (kernicterus) may cause sensory deficits cerebral palsy and mental retardation.

Box 11.4: Milestones of Development

Nothing on earth is more fascinating than watching a baby grow and develop. No two children are ever alike—not even twins in their growth and development and have individualistic patterns as variant and colorful like the views from a kaleidoscope. But there are some general principles. After birth and for the next several days the baby spends most of its time in sleeping. The motor movements are random and undirected (mass activity and reflexes). By about 2 weeks the baby smiles when touched (reflex smile) and tries to shift its body by kicking.

By the end of first month it tries to suck its thumb and can momentarily hold its head up while in a prone position. There are ocular pursuit movements. It continues to sleep most of the time but while awake waves the arms and legs. Cry becomes different when in pain and when hungry.

With the passage of another month the baby can momentarily fix its eyes on mother. Eyes follow bright objects. It can grasp a thing when put in its palm. It can also roll from side to back. By the third month its smiles at its mother and others who smile at him (social smile).

By the fourth month eye coordination is better. The eyes follow moving objects. Holds head in a sitting position. When lying down it turns from back to side. Reaches things with arms and grasp them. The baby is about 50 cm long now and weighs about 9 kg. It tries to pull its body into a sitting position. It sits with support and holds its head steadily by the fifth month. It grasps and holds things and makes cooing sounds.

When the baby is six months old and ready for the ritualistic rice feeding (annaprasana) ceremony it can roll about easily and can crawl around (prone body pulled by arms and legs). It smiles, laughs and plays with toes and makes hitching movements (moving backward in a sitting position).

Within the next 2–3 months the baby sits without support and creeps on hand and knees. It picks up objects with the thumb apposed. It can talk one or two syllables (babbling) and is able to stand with support.

By the time it celebrates its first birthday the baby creeps easily on all four limbs. It can now stand without support and walk with support. It has cut 4–6 teeth by now and is about 70 cm tall. It gazes at mirror and pictures, understands the meaning of yes or no and can speak 2–3 words. It tries to take food using figures. It can pick up small things and can pull itself to a standing position.

By one and half years the baby walks without support. Throws a ball; drinks from a cup or glass. Vocabulary consists of 4–5 words.

Bowel control is achieved by the 2nd year. It runs, climbs on a stool and balances on one foot. It has 16 teeth by now and is about 85 cm tall. It helps to wash and dress himself. Speech is clearer and it talks short sentences. It names familiar objects and can copy a circle.

By the 3rd year he (no more a baby but a toddler) can run quickly; has bladder control and rides tricycles. He points to all familiar things. Buttons and unbuttons his cloth. He is also ready to play with other children.

And the growth and development continues.

Postnatal Factors

Infections (encephalitis, meningitis, etc.) head injuries and epilepsy are some among the main postnatal factors of mental retardation. Poverty, malnutrition and an intellectually non-stimulating environment are other factors.

MANAGEMENT

Drugs have no role except in controlling associated physical or psychiatric conditions, as for example, when the child is violent or aggressive or destructive. Children who are severely or profoundly retarded may need institutionalization as constant nursing care may be needed. Children who are not violent or destructive may be nursed at home. Children who are educable (mild mental retardation) and trainable (moderate mental retardation) will benefit from special schools and training institutions. The National Institute for Mentally Retarded situated at Hyderabad, provides useful literature in training and rehabilitation of the mentally retarded.

Prophylactic measures are of great importance. In known cases of genetic predisposition genetic counseling should be given.

Proper antenatal, perinatal and postnatal care are also important. Many inborn errors of metabolism can be detected early and managed properly (as for example, withdrawing food containing phenylalanine in PKU). An emotionally and intellectually stimulating environment is essential for conductive growth.

Treatments in Psychiatry

Methods of treatment in psychiatry are sometimes divided into two groups:

1. Methods which are directly applied to the patient's body, these being invasive (meaning invading the body tissues) and known as the somatic or physical methods of treatment.

2. Those which are not invasive, known as the psychosocial methods.

PHYSICAL METHODS OF TREATMENT

These are mainly three:

1. Drugs

2. Electroconvulsive therapy (ECT)

3. Psychosurgery. Either temporary or permanent changes in the body are brought about by their use resulting in a cure or remission of symptoms.

DRUGS IN PSYCHIATRY

Drugs are psychopharmacological agents and are indicated in psychiatry: (a) to relieve pain and distress, (b) to bring about tranquility, (c) to promote sleep, (d) to control psychotic symptoms, (e) to elevate mood and (f) to stabilize mood. They are classified accordingly:

1. Drugs which relieve anxiety and distress (anxiolytics).

2. Drugs which promote sleep (hypnotics).

3. Drugs which control psychotic symptoms and produce tranquility (antipsychotics).

4. Drugs which elevate mood (mood elevators).
5. Drugs which stabilize the mood (mood stabilizers).
6. Other miscellaneous drugs.

Anxiolytics

Alcohol, bromides and opiates were used as anxiolytic medicines in the middle of 19th century. Barbiturates were introduced in the early 1900s as sedative-hypnotic drugs and were the first major anxiolytic drugs which were effective in reducing anxiety. Meprobamate, a carbamate derivative was introduced almost half a century later. Both barbiturates and meprobamate were disfavored because of their addictive property and lethality in high doses. Development and introduction of benzodiazepines in the 1960s were a major breakthrough. Azopyrones followed but unlike benzodiazepines they had a narrow spectrum of efficacy. Antidepressant drugs (tricyclic antidepressants in the 1960s and selective serotonin reuptake inhibitors in the 1990s — SSRI) were also used as anxiety relieving agents.

Meprobamate is a propanediol and was introduced as a muscle relaxant and sedative in 1956. It is an effective anti-anxiety agent. Drowsiness and dependence on long-term use are disadvantages.

Hydroxyzine is a diphenyl methane derivative and an antihistamine. It is a less potent anxiolytic drug. Other disadvantages are its rebound anxiety on withdrawal, drowsiness, dependence and respiratory depression.

Benzodiazepines

Several benzodiazepines are available for clinical use depending on their potency, plasma half lives and mode of action, this due to their specific receptor sites. The different receptor sites account for their anxiolytic, sedative and anticonvulsant properties. Most of the members act as hypnotics in higher doses. In spite of their high sedation they are nearer to an ideal anxiolytic drug.

They are absorbed easily though the oral route reaching the maximum plasma levels within 1–3 hours. Absorption is erratic through intramuscular route. They are lipophilic and cross the blood–brain barrier readily.

The anxiolytic benzodiazepines are divided into three subclasses depending on their structure: 2-keto (chlordiazepoxide, diazepam, clonazepam and the hypnotic flurazepam), 3-hydroxy (lorazepam, oxazepam) and triazo (alprazolam and the hypnotic triazolam).

Chlordiazepoxide is a long acting benzodiazepine with a half life of 14 hours after a single dose and up to 200 hours on repeated dosages due to the long half lives of its metabolites. It is an ideal drug in alcohol withdrawal states.

Diazepam has an action similar to chlordiazepoxide and is used in anxiety disorders, alcohol withdrawal states, for muscle relaxation and in convulsive disorders. It is rapidly absorbed and reaches plasma levels quickly. Being lipophilic it enters the brain readily.

Given intravenously it has an almost immediate action lasting for 20–30 minutes. It crosses the placenta, and is excreted in breast milk. Hypotonia and withdrawal symptoms may occur when used near delivery time. In the elderly diazepam may produce paradoxical reactions. Hypotension, muscle weakness, respiratory and cardiac arrest may occur with parenteral administration.

Lorazepam is a short acting benzodiazepine and has no active metabolites. It is less lipophilic than diazepam and produce clinical effects more slowly but provide more sustained relief.

Alprazolam and clonazepam are high potency benzodiazepines and are rapidly absorbed. Clinical effects appear within 30–60 minutes lasting for 8–12 hours. Both cross placental barrier and are excreted in breast milk.

Azaspirones

Buspirone is an example. It is less sedating than benzodiazepines and has antianxiety property. It is useful in general anxiety disorders (GAD) and is useful in the management of aggression in mental retardation. It has a low potential for abuse and withdrawal symptoms.

Some common anxiolytic drugs are listed in Table 12.1

Table 12.1: Some common anxiolytic drugs		
Drug	*Dose per day (mg)*	*Average elimination half life (hours)*
Alprazolam	1–4	12
Buspirone	15–30	10
Chlordiazepoxide	15–100	60–100
Clonazepam	1–4	36
Diazepam	10–60	60–100
Hydroxyzine	75–400	4
Lorazepam	2–10	12
Meprobamate	400–1200	8
Metoprolol	50–200	2–5
Oxazepam	30–120	10
Propranolol	40–120	2–5

Beta Blockers

Beta blockers are helpful in counteracting autonomic symptoms associated with anxiety, such as tremors and tachycardia. Metoprolol and propranolol are examples.

Hypnotics

Hypnotics are the drugs that induce sleep. Chloral hydrate and paraldehyde are some among the earliest drugs used to promote sleep but though safe are not prescribed because of their pungent odour, bad taste and gastric irritation. Short acting barbiturates and non-barbiturate agents like methaqualone and glutethimide are good hypnotics but are disfavored due to their abuse potential Table 12.2.

Benzodiazepines

Benzodiazepines are the most widely prescribed hypnotics and are relatively safe even in high dosage.

Flurazepam has a relatively long half life of about 40 hours. It has two active metabolites, one with a short half life and the other with a long half life. Because of these flurazepam induces sleep rapidly and sustain it for a long time. It is a safe hypnotic.

Nitrazepam is similar to flurazepam in having a rapid and prolonged action. It is also a safe hypnotic.

Triazolam has an extremely short half life (3–6 hours) and is rapidly absorbed (peak blood level within 20 minutes). It causes no daytime sedation.

Lorazepam is similar to nitrazepam and has a rapid onset of action. It has a higher abuse potential.

Other hypnotics — Nonbenzodiazepine hypnotics

Melatonin is a naturally occurring hormone produced by the pineal gland early during the sleep cycle possibly contributing to the natural circadian rhythm. It is helpful in mild insomnia and jet lag and is useful for the elderly.

L-tryptophan is an aminoacid free of dependence and abuse potential. It is useful in insomnia.

Zopiclone, zolpidem and zaleplon are nonbenzodiazepine hypnotics. Zopiclone is a short acting hypnotic compound which maintains sleep architecture. Zolpidem is an imidazopyrine with a short half life. Zaleplon is a pyrazoloprimidine and has a short half life. Unlike zolpidem zaleplon has muscle relaxant and anticonvulsant properties. Both are good inductors of sleep. Due to the short half life they do not produce a hang over effect.

ANTIPSYCHOTICS

Antipsychotics are also known as neuroleptics, psycholeptics and major tranquilizers. They differ from the other sedatives

Table 12.2: Some common hypnotics and their dosages	
Drug	*Dose*
Chloral hydrate	1–3 gm (orally)
Flurazepam	15–30 mg
Glutethimide	250–500 mg
Lorazepam	2–4 mg
Melatonin	2 mg
Methaqualone	150–300 mg
Nitrazepam	5–10 mg
Paraldehyde	2.5–5 gm (orally)
Triazolam	0.25–1 mg
L-tryptophan	1–5 gm
Zaleplon	5–10 mg
Zolpidem	5–10 mg
Zopiclone	3.75–10 mg

("minor tranquilizers") in several ways. Some differences are: (a) they cause sedation without inducing sleep, (b) control psychotic symptoms, agitation and excitement, (c) produce extrapyramidal symptoms and (d) they have a subcortical action. They are indicated therefore in conditions where there are psychotic symptoms like delusions, hallucinations and motor excitement (Table 12.3).

Phenothiazines

Chlorpromazine is probably the most well studied phenothiazine. It is a broad spectrum neuroleptic and has been used as a yard stick for other neuroleptic drugs. Pharmacologically it produces an "artificial hibernation"; it produces a sleep like state with indifference to surroundings. It decreases the aggressive behavior and increases sociability in animals and relieves the psychotic symptoms in man. It has antiemetic and hypotensive properties and causes hypothermia.

Trifluoperazine is some ten times more potent than chlorpromazine and produces more extrapyramidal symptoms.

Thioridazine is as effective as chlorpromazine but has lesser extrapyramidal symptoms.

Thioxanthenes

Chlorprothixene is the oldest member of thioxanthene group and is related in its clinical actions to chlorpromazine. In addition to antipsychotic properties it has antidepressant properties also

Table 12.3: Classification of antipsychotics

A. Phenothiazine derivatives
    i. Aliphatics (e.g. chlorpromazine)
    ii. Piperazines (e.g. trifluoperazine)
    iii. Piperidines (e.g. thioridazine)
B. Thioxanthine derivatives (e.g. flupenthixol)
C. Butyrophenon derivatives (e.g. haloperidol)
D. Diphenylbutylpiperidines (e.g. pimozide)
E. Others
    i. Benzamides (e.g. sulpiride)
    ii. Tricyclics (e.g. clozapine)
    iii. Dihydroindolone (e.g. malindone)

and is useful in agitation in depressed patients. The extra-pyramidal symptoms are less. It is safer in geriatric patients than chlorpromazine.

Butyrophenones

Though not chemically they are related to phenothiazines clinically. They are potent antipsychotics and cause less sedation. Extrapyramidal effects are more. *Haloperidol* is an example. In addition to psychosis haloperidol is useful in Tourette's disorder.

Diphenylbutylpiperidines

Structurally they are related to butyrophenones. *Pimozide* is an example. It is a potent antipsychotic and is particularly beneficial in delusional parasitosis.

Atypical Antipsychotics

The term "atypical antipsychotics" was coined in 1970 to denote a group of drugs which have largely supplanted the standard (typical) or conventional antipsychotics. They are preferred because of their low "side effect" profile and not because of their clinical efficiency. Extrapyramidal symptoms are minimal or absent and they are better than standard or typical antipsychotics in combating negative symptoms. There is no elevation of serum prolactin levels unlike typical ones and they have mood stabilizing or mood elevating properties in addition to antipsychotic effects.

Clozapine

Though synthesized in the 1960s its use was suspended in the 1970s following reported deaths due to agranulocytosis. It was reintroduced in 1988. It blocks various receptors powerfully—NA, 5-HT, histamine; ACh and DA receptors weakly. It blocks D_2 receptors least. There are no parkinsonian symptoms and dystonias or dyskinesias. In clinical efficacy it is superior to haloperidol or chlorpromazine and the drug is ideal in the treatment of refractory schizophrenias. About 1% of all patients on clozapine develop agranulocytosis which is not dose related but is believed to be an autoimmune reaction. Periodical blood counts are therefore necessary.

Risperidone is another atypical antipsychotic and is useful in both positive and negative symptoms. It causes minimal extrapyramidal symptoms.

Olanzapine is useful in positive and negative symptoms of schizophrenia. Like cloazapine it blocks several receptors. It is useful in post schizophrenic depression and in schizoaffective disorder. Somnolence and weight gain are common side effects.

Quetiapine has low affinity for D_2 receptors and extrapyramidal symptoms are minimal. It is comparable to standard antipsychotics in controlling positive symptoms but are more effective in treating negative symptoms. Somnolence and dizziness are common side effects.

Other atypical antipsychotics are ziprasidone and aripiprazole.

Adverse Effects of Antipsychotics

Pseudoparkinsonism
This is similar to parkinson's disease but pill rolling movements are rare. Muscles stiffness, cogwheel rigidity, stooped posture, mask like facies and drooling are common.

Dystonias
Painful muscle spasm of tongue, jaw and neck can develop in the first week of starting antipsychotic therapy. Acute dystonia may be terrifying. Opisthotonus of the whole body with extensor rigidity may occur.

Akathesia
This presents as restlessness and an urge to pace up and down or move from one position to another.

Parkinsonism, dystonia and akathesia are due to DA deficiency.

Tardive dyskinesia
Involuntary, irregular choreiform or athetoid movements may develop on prolonged (tardive = delayed) use of antipsychotics. These movements involve jaws (chewing) tongue (darting, twisting, protrusion) or fingers. Facial grimaces, torticollis or retrocollis, trunk twisting, athetoid arm and shoulder movements are other features which can be seen isolatedly or in combinations.

Neuroleptic Malignant Syndrome

Though rare the syndrome carries a high mortality and is characterized by ANS (autonomic nervous system) instability (fluctuating pulse rate, tachycardia and BP, hyperthermia, sweating) and muscular rigidity. Most cases develop within the first month, many within the first week.

The main side effects are listed in Table 12.4.

| **Table 12.4:** Major adverse effects of antipsychotic drugs ||
System	*Effects*
Neurological	
CNS	Pseudoparkinsonism, dystonia, akinesia, dyskinesias, akathesia
ANS	Urinary retention, orthostatic hypotension, failure to ejaculate, dry mount, visual blurring, constipation
Endocrine system	Amenorrhea, galactorrhea, loss of libido, impotence, weight gain
Cardiovascular system	Orthostatic hypotension, tachycardia, ECG changes
Others	Neuroleptic malignant syndrome, skin rashes, pigment deposits in the eye and skin, cholestatic jaundice

Table 12.5 shows the dosage schedules of the common antipsychotic drugs and their equivalence.

| **Table 12.5:** Antipsychotics—dosage and equivalence |||
Drug	*Average daily dose (mg)*	*Equivalence*
Chlorpromazine	100–300 (up to 1500)	100 mg
Clozapine	300–600	50 mg
Haloperidol	5–15 (up to 40)	5 mg
Olanzapine	5–20	5 mg
Quetiapine	300–500	—
Risperidone	2–6 (up to 10)	1 mg
Thioridazine	100–300 (up to 800)	100 mg
Trifluoperazine	5–30 (up to 60)	5 mg
Ziprasidone	60–120	—

Antidepressants

Antidepressants are the drugs that elevate mood and relieve depression. They should be differentiated from psycho-stimulants like amphetamine. Psychostimulants have no antidepressant effect but instead produce a temporary euphoric effect by direct stimulation of the brain. Further, euphoria is followed by a rebound depression when the former effects wear off.

Tricyclic Antidepressants

Imipramine was the first compound synthesized in 1957 and its antidepressant property was an accidental discovery. Other members of this category are trimipramine, nortripty-line, amytriptyline, dothiepin, etc. They are safe and cheap antidepressants. They act by increasing the availability of monoamines in the synaptic cleft by blocking their reuptake.

Monoamine Oxidase (MAO) Inhibitors

Monoamines are oxidased by the enzyme monoamine oxidase in the synaptic cleft. By inhibiting this enzyme the concentration of monoamines is enhanced. MAO inhibitors act in this manner. When food containing tyramine (present in cheese, broad bears, etc.) is taken simultaneously toxic complications (hypertensive crises) occur. Therefore, they are to be used with caution. Phenelzine and niamid are the examples of this group.

SSRI and SNRI

SSRI (Serotonin specific reuptake inhibitors) selectively block reuptake of serotonin and SNRI (Serotonin norepine-phrine reuptake inhibitors) block serotonin and norepine-phrine. Fluoxetine and venlafaxine are respective examples. Some common antidepressants are listed in Table 12.6.

Adverse Effects

CNS: Dizziness, ataxia, tremors, seizures.
ANS: Dryness of mouth, blurred vision, urinary retention, constipation.

Table 12.6: Common antidepressants and their dosage

Drug	Average daily dose (mg)
Amytriptyline	75–150 mg
Clomipramine	75–150 mg
Dothiepin	100–300 mg
Doxepin	100–200 mg
Fluoxetine	20–60 mg
Fluvoxamine	50–200 mg
Imipramine	75–150 mg
Mianserin	30–120 mg
Nortriptyline	75–150 mg
Phenelzine	30–90 mg
Sertraline	50–200 mg
Trimipramine	75–150 mg
Venlafaxine	75–300 mg

CVS: Postural hypotension, tachycardia.

GI: Cholestasis.

Haematological: Agranulocytosis

Dermatological: Skin rashes.

Endocrine: Weight gain, amenorrhea, gynecomastia, sexual disturbances.

Mood Stabilizers

Mood stabilizers are the drugs that have a prophylactic role in both manic and depressive cycles of a bipolar disorder. The first drug of this category was lithium after its discovery in 1949 of having such properties. Later other members were added to the list namely, valproate, carbamazepine, lamotrigine, gabapentin, topiramate and tiagabine.

Lithium

Lithium salts were used in gout as early as 1817 but its psychiatric uses were discovered by Cade in 1949 only. It controls symptoms of acute mania and is effective in reducing recurrences of both bipolar and unipolar affective disorders. Lithium is most commonly available as carbonate but citrate and acetate forms are also available. These also are equally effective.

Lithium has a narrow safety margin and serum concentrations are to be frequently monitored. Blood drawn 12 hours after the last dose is used for the serum level estimation. A serum level of 0.8–1.2 mEq/L is considered adequate and this level is usually obtained by oral doses of 600–1500 mg lithium per day. Higher blood levels cause toxic symptoms to appear. These include coarse tremors, ataxia, confusion, muscular weakness, seizures, anorexia, vomiting, polyuria, polydipsia and ECG changes. Lithium induces nontoxic goiter and produces acne and exacerbation of psoriasis.

Sodium Valproate

Valproate is available in various forms — as valproic acid, sodium valproate, divalproex sodium and a combination of valproic acid and sodium valproate. Valproate is converted to valproic acid in the stomach and totally absorbed from the gestrointestinal tract.

Valproate is equally effective as lithium in acute mania and in the prophylaxis of bipolar disorder. It is particularly effective in rapid cycling mood disorders (more than four cycles per year) for which it is the preferred drug. It is effective in the treatment of agitation, aggression and impulsivity of bipolar disorders. The usual daily dose is 400–600 mg which may be increased to 1600 mg/day. Plasma levels do not correlate with therapeutic efficacy. Nausea and vomiting are the commonest adverse effects. Others are tiredness, tremors, alopecia and jaundice.

Carbamazepine

Carbamazepine was synthesized in 1957 and introduced as an antiepileptic. Due to its structural similarity to imipramine it was used as an antidepressant. Its use in acute mania and in bipolar disorders was later confirmed either alone or along with lithium and valproate. It is superior to lithium in rapid cycling bipolar disorders. The daily dosage may range from 400 to 1600 mg in divided doses. Sedation, ataxia, gastric irritation and drug rashes are adverse effects which are commonly encountered. Though rare a serious adverse effect is thrombocytopenia, agranulocytosis and aplastic anemia.

Lamotrigine

Lamotrigine is an anticonvulsant indicated in partial complex and generalized seizures but has in addition mood stabilizing properties. The effects are attributed to modulation of reuptake of serotonin and monoamines including dopamine. It has found use in bipolar and unipolar depression, cyclothymia and schizoaffective disorder. It is well tolerated at doses of 50–200 mg per day stepped up in small increment of 25 mg once in 3–4 days. Weakness, diplopia, headache, nausea and ataxia are the usual side effects.

Miscellaneous Drugs

Antiparkinsonian Drugs

Treatment with neuroleptics is almost always associated with extrapyramidal symptoms. They are mainly of four types:

1. Pseudoparkinsonism (rigidity, tremors, akinesia and loss of associate movements).
2. Dystonia (dyskinesia, torticollis, torsion dystonias).
3. Akathesia (mental and motor restlessness. Restless legs syndrome).
4. Tardive dyskinesia (choreoathetoid movements of hands and shoulders, chewing movements, tongue darting, etc.).

Drugs commonly used in the above conditions are listed in Table 12.7.

Table 12.7: Drugs used in the treatment of extrapyramidal symptoms

Drugs	Dose	Indications
Anticholinergics		
Benztropine	Tab 0.5 mg tds	Dystonia, akathesia, parkinsonism
Diphenylhydramine	Tab 2.5 mg tds	- do -
Procyclidine	Tab 2.5 mg tds	Dystonia, parkinsonism
Trihexyphenidyl	Tab 2 mg tds	- do -
Betablockers		
Propranolol	Tab 20 mg tds	Akathesia
Dopamine agonists		
Amantidine	Tab 100 mg bid	Akinesia, parkinsonism
Bromocriptine	Tab 1.2 mg bid	Neuroleptic malignant syndrome
Antidopaminergics	Tab 1 mg bid	Tardive dyskinesia

CONVULSIVE THERAPIES

The convulsive therapies originated with a mistaken belief that epilepsy did not coexist with mental illness. Further in epileptic patients psychiatric symptoms at times improved after a seizure. With this belief attempts were made to produce artificial convulsions as a method of treatment of psychiatric illness. Von Meduna in 1933 used 25% camphor in oil which he injected intramuscularly. 10–40 ml oil (2.5–10 ml of camphor) had to be injected to produce a convulsion which was unpredictable with respect to the time of onset of convulsions. Also it was a terrifying experience for the patient till he lost consciousness. This led to the choice of a soluble synthetic camphor preparation, pentamethylentetrazol (Metrazol or Cardiazol) given as a 10% solution. The convulsions set in between 5 and 30 seconds after the injection which also had the disadvantage as above—failure to produce a convulsion needing a repeated dose, and apprehension and discomfort till he lost consciousness.

In 1938, Cerletti and Bini, two Italian psychiatrists used electric current to produce convulsions and a new method of treatment called electroconvulsive therapy (ECT) came into being. It had the advantages of being simpler, cleaner and safer than the pharmacological convulsion therapies. The patient lost consciousness almost instantaneously as the current was applied and there was no apprehension or discomfort. This led to the preferential use of ECT to pharmacological convulsion therapies.

In 1957, Krantz and his coworkers while studying some fluorinated ethers came across a compound, hexafluorodiethyl ether (Indoklon) which in smaller concentrations produced (20–30 parts to a million in the inspired air) convulsions and higher doses (6–8% of air) produced anesthesia. It is a colorless noninflammable liquid which is applied by means of a mask and a vaporizer. The convulsion occurred within 15–30 seconds. The disadvantage is the inability to judge whether the patient had an optimal convulsion as some myoclonic movements preceded the convulsion and often replaced it.

Electroconvulsive Therapy (ECT)

It is customary nowadays to give "modified" ECT as described below which is preferable to the "unmodified" (or direct) ECT because of its several advantages. The muscular contractions in direct ECT are strong and often painful after the ECT.

Preparation of the Patient

The patient should be starving for 6–8 hours prior to ECT. On the morning of the treatment atropine (0.5–1 mg) is given intramuscularly to dry throat secretions and to prevent vagally mediated bronchospasm, bradyarrhythmias and asystole. The patient is asked to empty bladder. If clothings are worn tightly they are loosened. Sharp objects like safety pins, hairpins and slides are removed as well as artificial denture, contact lenses, spectacles, hearing aids, etc. if patient is wearing them.

Administration of ECT

100–200 mg of 10% pentothal sodium (or any other ultra short acting barbiturates) is given as a 10% solution followed by a muscle relaxant like succinyl chloride (scoline 20–40 mg) both intravenously. Since succinylcholine paralyses respiratory muscles also respiration is maintained by mechanical means. Patient should be oxygenated. The skin in the temples on both sides is cleaned and a conducting jelly is applied. Electrical stimulus is delivered by the electrodes bilaterally which results in instantaneous loss of consciousness and tonic clonic seizures lasting for 30–60 seconds. Patient is transferred to the recovery room after the convulsions are over and patient starts to breath spontaneously.

Observation in the Recovery Room

Respiration, pulse and BP are recorded and patient is watched against prolonged seizures, excitement and vomiting (danger of aspiration) when patient is fully awake he may be transferred to the wards.

In the direct ECT barbiturates and scoline are not given. Electrical stimulus is applied directly to the two temples bilaterally. In unilateral ECT stimulus is applied only on one side (nondominant side) of the brain.

ECT is indicated in depression, particularly when it is associated with agitation or psychotic symptoms, some types of schizophrenia (catatonic and paranoid), in schizophrenic and depressive stupors and some types of delirium. It is not given in neuroses. ECT should not be given after a recent myocardial infarction and in space occupying lesions of the brain or in hemorrhage. ECT is usually a safe procedure and there are no adverse effects except for temporary, but recoverable amnesia. In pathological conditions (e.g. osteoporosis) the strong convulsions may lead to fracture of the bone unless ECT is suitably modified.

PSYCHOSOCIAL METHODS OF TREATMENT

The physical or somatic methods of treatment are referred to as invasive methods, meaning they invade or penetrate the body tissues producing changes in them. On the contrary, psychosocial methods are noninvasive in nature. There are several types of psychosocial methods of treatment but the main ones are the various forms of psychotherapy, behaviour therapy and the occupational and recreational therapies.

Box 12.1: Occupational Therapy

Mooted with the idea that "an idle mind is the devil's workshop" it was recognized that mental patients also, like normal people need to be constantly engaged to be free from monotony and boredom. This corresponded in time to the "humane reforms" (removal of chains that bound patients, etc.) and was then known as moral treatment.

However, it is not in this narrow sense—as providing an alternate task to fill an idle moment—that occupational therapy is envisaged in modern times. It aids physical and psychological rehabilitation. To this end activities are carefully selected and a particular activity best suited for a specific psychopathological state is prescribed. The earlier forms of activity like walking, games, etc. are supplemented with crafts, painting, music, dance, sculpture, reading, etc. Art is a powerful mode of self expression. Patient's artistic productions often give insight into their problems. Patients are encouraged to explain their paintings or sculptures which aid treatment.

Occupational therapy adds to the patient's resources and helps them to adopt to their physical and psychological needs: (i) its own merit, (ii) by being complementary to other forms of treatment and 3. by its utility not only during the time of treatment but even after recovery.

Psychotherapies

An effective theraupetic relationship between patient and the doctor underlies all forms of treatment. But the term psycho-therapy is restricted to the methods of "alleviation of personal distress through the medium of words in a professional setting". There are over a hundred forms of psychotherapy which differ from each other in the way of conducting them, their therapeutic set up and theoretical foundations.

Psychotherapies differ in other aspects also—like the number of participants at a time, length of treatment period and the depth of exploration. In individual psychotherapy only one patient (some times called the client) is engaged at a time whereas in group therapy treatment is provided to a group of people simultaneously. Again, the group may be small (5-8 members) or large (20–50 members). The group may be homo-geneous (e.g. drug addicts alone, adolescents, homosexuals, etc.) or not (heterogeneous collection of an array of problems). Some forms of psychotherapy continue for several months or even years whereas some others are of a short duration, extending to a few sessions only. In deep psycho-therapy the underlying conflicts are explored more intensively and worked through in great detail which is not done in supportive forms of therapy. In supportive forms of therapy the person's existing coping skills are utilized to tide over the crisis. The patient is helped to achieve his best level of functioning through emotional support, guidance and counseling. In the deep therapy newer and more effective coping mechanisms are sought to be adaptive by the patient.

Another way of classifying the psychotherapies is by categorizing them as: (i) supportive, (ii) re-educative and (iii) re-constructive. The supportive forms as mentioned earlier aims at promoting and reinforcing the patient's existing potentials. Reassurance, motivation, guidance, persuasion, etc. belong to this category. In re-educative therapies the patient is given better insight into his problems. He is educated on the need of modifying his goals and means of achieving them by using his existing skills. Counseling, reconditioning attitude changing, etc. belong to this class of treatment. In reconstructive therapies the patient is given deeper and fuller understanding on the nature of the conflict. He is encouraged to extensively alter his character and coping skills. The various forms of psychodynamic psychotherapies belong to this category.

Indications

Psychotherapy is indicated in neurotic disorders and mild personality disorders, in people who are motivated and who are reasonably intelligent. To benefit from the treatment the patient should be able to understand what is told to him and should also be able to verbalize and communicate his problems. It is not the primary line of treatment in psychotic disorders, severe personality disorders and heavy dependence on drugs.

Individual Psychotherapy

As mentioned above there are different forms of individual psychotherapy depending on the theoretical basis, methods of conducting them and the depth of exploration.

Psychoanalysis

Formulated by Sigmund Freud, psychoanalysis is a form of treatment and also a method of investigating mental processes, based on the principles of psychoanalytic psychology. Mention was made about these principles in the chapter on neurotic disorders. It is dynamic and interpretative in nature and uses *"free association"* as a method to bring out the repressed material to conscious awareness. Fifty minute sessions numbering 3–5 times per week are held for several months or years.

Supportive Psychotherapy

Supportive psychotherapy is a non-exploratory form of psychological treatment and involves discussion of the patient's problems at a simple pragmatic level. The therapist provides emotional support and advice. The therapy is limited to a few sessions with provision for more sessions when need arises. This can be combined with the physical methods of treatment. Medicines are given to patients who need them.

Counseling

Counseling is a form of re-educative type of psychotherapy and is given to people having relationship or adjustment problems, as for example, family members, marital partners, etc. in vocational, familial or other settings like schools.

Group Therapy

When two or more patients participate in the treatment at the same time it forms a group. In addition to the small–large and homogeneous–heterogeneous differentiation of groups (mentioned earlier), there is another important distinction in the group structure—the open *vs.* the closed group. In the former, all members start treatment at the same time and continue together till the group is dissolved. The number of participants remain the same unless a member drops out. He may be replaced by a new member or not as decided by the group. In the open group members are allowed to terminate treatment and leave in the middle and new members are allowed to join the group at any time. Groups also differ depending on the treatment modality and the role of the therapist during the sessions—his taking the role of a passive catalyst or by actively exploring an interpreting the data.

Group therapy is more powerful than individual psycho-therapy at least to some patients. Therapeutic effects occur more readily in the group and are more sustained. The group itself is the main therapeutic agent in group therapy unlike in individual psychotherapy. The factors which affect a cure are:

1. Patient's sense of group belonginess and commitment.
2. Chances to learn from others' behavior.
3. Universality—or an understanding that he is not the lone sufferer and that.
4. There are others who have the similar problems.
5. Hopefulness which is enhanced when he sees improvement in other members of the group.
6. **Modelling:** Adopting new coping skills shown by other group members which he perceives are helpful for himself.

Behavior Therapies

Behaviour therapies are based on assumptions of the behavior theory that all behavior, adaptive or non-adaptive are learnt responses. Neurotic symptoms are the result of faulty learning. What is learnt is amenable to "unlearning". As per the learning theory such maladaptive responses can be inhibited or extinguished by certain techniques which are advocated in behavior therapies. Psychogenesis of symptoms is irrelevant according to behavior theories. Instead of psychodynamic factors objective observable behavior is accessible to correction leading to a cure.

Box 12.2: Pavlov and Conditioning

Ivan Pavlov, the Russian physiologist famous for his conditioning studies on dogs postulated that when a "neutral" stimulus is coupled with a "natural" stimulus, the former over a course of time behaves like the natural stimulus. To illustrate sound of a bell is coupled with the sight of food. After a few trials the animal responded to the sound of the bell in a manner similar to the sight of food, i.e. by salivation. The bell is the neutral stimulus and food the natural stimulus. Salivation is the natural response when food is sighted. Pavlov rang the bell each time the dog was given food. Over the course of time the dogs started salivating at the sound of the bell in anticipation of food. After conditioning the bell is known as the conditioned stimulus and salivation the conditioned response. The process by which the neutral stimulus becomes the conditioned stimulus is known as conditioning. This is an example of substitute learning, the bell being the substitute for food. To represent the process schematically

Ringing of bell (neutral stimulus)	$\longrightarrow$	No salivation
Sight of food (natural stimulus)	$\longrightarrow$	Salivation (natural response)
Bell + Food	$\longrightarrow$	Salivation (conditioning)
Bell alone (conditioned stimulus)	$\longrightarrow$	Salivation (conditioned response)

This form of conditioning is known as classical (Pavlovian conditioning). Some concepts related to classical conditioning are:

1. *Generalization*: Stimuli resembling the original stimulus will evoke the same response.
2. *Reinforcement*: Each time bell is coupled (given along) with food the response (salivation) is reinforced
3. *Extinction*: When food is not given along with bell, after some time the response (salivation) *extinguishes* (disappears)
4. *Reconditioning*: The behavior can be re-established when bell is again coupled with food. In addition to the classical conditioning there are other variant forms of conditioning. A good deal of human learning follows the principles of conditioning. Also they provide the foundations for behavior therapy

The techniques used in behavior therapy include desensitization, aversion therapy, stimulus flooding, conditioning, assertive training, biofeedback, etc.

Cognitive Therapy

While behavior therapy is based on the assumption that maladaptive behavior is the cause of one's faulty perceptions and thinking (cognitions) about oneself and the world around him there is another form of therapy founded on the belief that abnormal cognitions are the cause and not the result of maladaptive behavior. As for example, depression is the result of one's distorted view of himself as a derogatory figure. Treatment is aimed at altering the cognitions through verbal means (explanation, discussion, etc.) or by using techniques of behavior therapy. Therefore, cognitive therapy is sometimes called as cognitive behavior therapy (CBT).

Box 12.3: Psychodrama
Psychodrama essentially is a form of group therapy conducted inside the wards of a hospital. It was originally created by Moreno in 1912, but underwent several modifications by the later therapists. The intended purpose is to encourage patients express their feelings by taking up different roles along with other patient actors on the stage. Those who are not participating as well as the staff form the audience. After a scene is enacted the audience is asked to make comments or to interrupt what they have observed. Psychodrama is based on the assumption that actions or dramatic representations are more eloquent than verbal presentation of one's problems. In psychodrama the responses are more spontaneous. It also facilitates total perception of one's unhealthy responses and the impediments in tackling them in real life.

Other methods of psychosocial methods of treatment are occupational and recreational therapy, psychodrama, hypnosis, music therapy, bibliotherapy, yoga therapy, etc.

Index